NATURE AND NURTURE IN MENTAL DISORDERS

A GENE-ENVIRONMENT MODEL

Second Edition

NATURE AND NURTURE IN MENTAL DISORDERS

A GENE-ENVIRONMENT MODEL

Second Edition

Joel Paris, M.D.
Professor Emeritus of Psychiatry, McGill University,
Montreal, Quebec, Canada

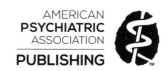

AMERICAN
PSYCHIATRIC
ASSOCIATION
PUBLISHING

American Psychiatric Association Publishing
800 Maine Avenue SW
Suite 900
Washington, DC 20024-2812
www.appi.org

Library of Congress Cataloging-in-Publication Data
Names: Paris, Joel, author.
Title: Nature and nurture in mental disorders : a gene-environment model / Joel Paris.
Other titles: Nature and nurture in psychiatry
Description: Second edition. | Washington, DC : American Psychiatric Association Publishing, [2021] | Preceded by: Nature and nurture in psychiatry : a predisposition-stress model of mental disorders / by Joel Paris. Washington, DC : American Psychiatric Press, Inc., c1999. | Includes bibliographical references and index.
Identifiers: LCCN 2020033272 (print) | LCCN 2020033273 (ebook) | ISBN 9781615373345 (paperback) alk. paper | ISBN 9781615373680 (ebook)
Subjects: MESH: Mental Disorders—genetics | Mental Disorders—psychology | Genetic Predisposition to Disease | Stress, Psychological | Models, Psychological
Classification: LCC RC455.4.G4 (print) | LCC RC455.4.G4 (ebook) | NLM WM 140 | DDC 616.89/042—dc23
LC record available at https://lccn.loc.gov/2020033272
LC ebook record available at https://lccn.loc.gov/2020033273

British Library Cataloguing in Publication Data
A CIP record is available from the British Library.

Contents

Part III
Implications

━━ PREFACE TO THE SECOND EDITION

THE FIRST edition of this book was published in 1999. That year marked the end of the "decade of the brain." Over the next two decades, neuroscience continued to advance and has become the primary basis of clinical work. Yet, in many ways, we just do not know enough to practice on the basis of neuroscience. Some claim that research will lead to personalized medicine based on individual differences in the genome, but that is not likely to happen anytime soon.

Nineteen ninety-eight was a time when many of us anticipated that the decoding of the genome would lead to dramatic scientific breakthroughs. As far as both medicine and psychiatry were concerned, however, we were wrong. This new edition of the book draws on genomewide association studies to show that most human traits are influenced by hundreds if not thousands of genes. This level of complexity means it will be many decades before genetics can be applied to understanding and treating mental disorders.

We should keep in mind that it is early days for neuroscience, and findings could eventually lead to more treatment options. Yet an equally strong literature supports the importance of environmental risk factors in mental disorders. This book shows that, for most conditions seen in psychiatry, both genes and environment play a major role in etiology.

Most of the previous edition of this book is now out of date; thus, the second edition has been almost entirely rewritten. This new version shows how current evidence supports an interactive model, combining recent data from neuroscience with a large body of evidence about the influence of the psychosocial environment. I have therefore changed the subtitle of the book from "predisposition-stress" to the more precise "gene-environment" model. In the first edition, I focused concern about reliance on overly environmental models of psychopathology, particularly those based on psychoanalysis or on narrowly based sociocultural theories. But those ideas have undergone a steady decline. Over the past 20 years, psychiatry has become much more biological in orientation. I now see a different set of problems, with the greater danger now lying in ignoring the environment entirely.

We hear the common mantra that "mental disorders are brain disorders." There is, of course, no such thing as mind without brain—they are just different levels of looking at human thought, emotion, and behavior. But I disagree with reducing the mind, which has crucial emergent properties, to the level of neuronal function. I also disagree with the idea that the complexity of mental illnesses, from the most severe to the most common, can be fully explained at a cellular or neurochemical level. That narrow vision helps explain why so many patients today, particularly those diagnosed with depression, are being treated entirely with medication. This kind of practice is based on the idea that mental disorders can be entirely accounted for by abnormalities in neurotransmission or neuroconnectivity.

This second edition argues that this reductionistic view is not supported by firm evidence. Instead, it supports a biopsychosocial model in which the object of study is the mind and the person. It rejects both biological and psychosocial reductionism; instead, the link between mind and brain is best accounted for by gene-environment interactions. When one thinks interactively, a nature-nurture dichotomy becomes unnecessary.

These ideas are hardly original; most clinicians would agree with them in principle. However, the biopsychosocial model is often paid lip service and not taken seriously. The result is a practice in which clinicians replace understanding of life experience with DSM-based checklists and overly zealous pharmacological interventions. Another message of this book is that a broader model has important clinical implications. Genes and environment need to be studied—not separately, but in interaction. Based on a large body of research conducted over the past 20 years, combining neuroscience with social sciences could become the basis of more effective treatment.

Unfortunately, the divide between the "two cultures" of psychiatry continues to interfere with progress in planning treatment. Researchers in neuroscience may either ignore effects of the environment or measure them with vague concepts such as "stress" or "trauma." At the same time, although researchers on the psychosocial factors in mental disorders may know that half the variance affecting psychopathology is genetic, they apply models that allow them to ignore this fact. Few studies measure both genetic and environmental risk factors in the same populations. With some significant exceptions, neuroscience and developmental psychopathology have not found a common meeting place.

The human mind is programmed to look for simple and direct relationships between cause and effect. Clinicians, like the rest of us, have trouble with complexities. What can be hard to grasp is that no single or simple risk factors for most forms of psychopathology have been identified. A theory based on interacting multiple risk factors, taking into account large numbers of genes as well as multiple interacting environmental stressors, is needed to address these problems.

▬ INTRODUCTION

HUMANITY IS a single species. All of us share most of our 20,000+ genes and have the same body plan as well as similar mental patterns. These similarities are driven by natural selection. Yet at the same time, people are very different from each other. Any theory of mental disorders must account for both similarities and differences. What is the source of individual variability? Some of these differences are also shaped by natural selection. The genes that drive individual differences may be in the minority, but they have profound effects. Each reflects an adaptation to an historical or current environment or a range of traits than can cope with different environmental circumstances. Thus, humans differ in physical characteristics, such as height, facial features, and skin color. We are also mentally different—in our thoughts, our emotions, and our behaviors.

Physical differences have always been understood as related to genetic influence. However, mental differences have not always been seen in the same light. Over the centuries, philosophers and scientists have struggled with the *nature-nurture problem*. In other words, are we more a product of our genes or of our environment?

Even if the answer is "both," this issue remains the center of intense controversy. For example, clinicians and researchers continue to debate the extent to which clinical depression derives from a chemical imbalance or whether lowered mood is largely a response to loss and disappointment. Similar debates have raged over the origins of other mental disorders, but as psychiatry moved back to its roots in medicine, it became more biological and tended to favor nature over nurture.

This dichotomy has played an important role in psychiatric practice. When I was a resident, nurture was often favored over nature. One of my teachers, a psychoanalyst who headed a hospital department, was sympathetic to attempts to cure schizophrenia with psychotherapy. When I suggested that this was not a reasonable goal for a disorder that was strongly genetic, he became angry, stating, "I will not see patients as incurable and let them go down the drain." Years later, he changed his mind after reading a landmark study showing that psychotherapy is not effective for the management of acute psychoses (May 1968).

Psychotherapists who believe that everything problematic in life derives from childhood adversities and inadequate parenting tend to have a utopian vision of what mental health treatment can accomplish. This is why they, all too often, see patients for years, hoping to achieve the impossible. Biological psychiatrists are more likely to think that, until we learn how to rewrite the genome, there will always be constraints on how much people can change. Yet they too tend to chase impossible outcomes, usually by prescribing too many drugs. An interactive model can help us to come to terms with our limitations.

These clinical problems are also reflected in the research community, in which neuroscience ignores the environment while psychology ignores genetics. Future research needs to integrate nature and nurture and use measures of both in the same populations. Although that program is in a very early stage, psychiatrists of the future will eventually benefit from knowing more precisely how genes and environment interact to produce mental disorders.

THE ORIGINS OF THIS BOOK

This book has both intellectual and personal roots. One of my motivations in writing this second edition is to summarize what I have learned in 50 years as a psychiatrist. At the same time, I want to share with readers what I have had to *unlearn*. When I began my training in the 1960s, there was not much contact between strains of thought that favored nature or nurture. They ran in parallel without ever meeting. Like many North American residents at that time, I had psychoanalysts as teachers who believed that the causes of common mental disorders lie in an unhappy childhood. Their models were seductive because they offered an understanding of almost every form of psychopathology, but these ideas were inaccurate and simplistic.

At the same time, psychiatry was in the midst of a psychopharmacological revolution. In the most severe disorders, drugs were usually superior to psychotherapy. Moreover, drugs were starting to be applied to patients who were symptomatic but less impaired. I could not anticipate that millions of patients would be taking psychiatric drugs, sometimes for a lifetime. A new paradigm has replaced a biopsychosocial mode (Engel 1980) with what, among others, Bentall (2009) has called a "bio-bio-bio" model.

I have never disagreed with the principle that mental disorders are brain disorders. Of course they are! However, that does not mean that thoughts, behaviors, and emotions are best understood by reduction to a neuronal level. Moreover, a biopsychosocial model leads to different clinical implications. For a good number of patients, ranging from those with mild depression to those with a personality disorder, medication is of doubtful value and psychotherapy is the treatment of choice. For others, a combination of drugs and talking therapy is the best option.

When I began to practice psychiatry, I wanted to justify my years of training in medicine and treat patients who were sick enough to require the services of a physician. I was particularly interested and challenged by patients who were chronically suicidal. These patients were often avoided by nonmedical clinicians, and if, by the end of treatment, they decided to go on living, I would know that they had benefited. This is why I became interested in the treatment of borderline personality disorder. At the time, a psychodynamic model seemed to have the most to offer, and that is what I offered my patients in the early years of my career. Like most clinicians, I started with high hopes but achieved mixed results. Some patients did brilliantly—these are the cases clinicians like to write up and talk about. Other patients deteriorated in spite of my best efforts. Most showed middling levels of improvement.

I also took a psychodynamic perspective as a teacher of psychiatric residents. Whatever the presenting problems, I could come up with a plausible explanation based on the patient's personal history. I later came to the conclusion that this way of thinking was specious, and I began to adopt a hardheaded approach based on empirical evidence. I came to consider myself a "born-again" proponent of evidence-based practice. I have wondered if I should undertake a "product recall" and inform residents from the 1970s to ignore my earlier views, but my students have almost certainly forgotten most of what I taught them.

In the course of a long career, my ideas about psychiatry have changed dramatically. For nearly 50 years, I have been in charge of an outpatient consultation clinic evaluating a large number of new patients referred from the community. I have now seen about 50,000 cases—approximately the population of a small town. Exposure to a very broad range of psychopathology helped me to appreciate the complexity of the pathways to mental illness. I benefit, at least in principle, from this experience. However, as this book argues, clinical experience is not a reliable guide to understanding causes. Like any scientific hypothesis, intuitive impressions need to be confirmed by systematic research.

I have been fortunate to have colleagues who helped me to develop a second career as a researcher. In spite of my late arrival on the scientific scene, beginning as a clinician-teacher had some advantages. My experiences led me to address the question as to why some patients develop one type of illness under adverse circumstances while other patients, faced with the same life events, develop a completely different type of illness, and still others develop no illness at all. My own research has focused on patients who do not benefit from standard treatments. This lack of response requires an explanation. Traditionally, clinicians believed that the intractability of personality disorders derived from their roots in early childhood. However, research does not confirm this view and shows that most people who experience early adversities never develop a mental disorder (Paris 2020). Life events alone do not account for the development of personality disorders or, for that matter, of most mental disorders.

Several lines of evidence, described in detail in this book, support this conclusion (Cicchetti 2016). Many patients with mental disorders have no history of childhood adversity. Patients with similar life experiences can develop completely different illnesses. Children experiencing severe adversities show high levels of resilience, and only a minority will develop diagnosable psychopathology in adulthood. Moreover, children raised in the same family and exposed to the same environment do not necessarily have the same outcome as adults. Finally, research in behavior genetics shows that about half of the variance affecting most mental disorders is genetic (Plomin 2018).

Psychopathology in any individual is not predictable, either from inborn temperament alone or from life experience by itself. The problem with current models in psychiatry is that they heavily tilt the scales, one way or the other, toward genes or environment. The biomedical model attempts to view psychopathology as entirely a function of abnormal neuroconnectivity or neurochemistry. In doing so, it radically oversimplifies the complexity of the human brain and mind. This model works best for psychoses, as well as neurodevelopmental disorders and neurocognitive disorders, but even there has limitations.

A purely psychological or psychosocial model of psychopathology is equally simplistic and misleading. When events in an individual's life have been adverse, it may seem plausible to account for present difficulties by personal history. However, what clinicians do not always realize is that their patients are a highly selected subsample of those exposed to any given risk factor. When researchers go out into the community and interview nonclinical samples, they find that most people exposed to negative life events develop mild difficulties or none at all.

These facts are striking. To explain them, we need a different and more interactive theoretical model, one that integrates nature and nurture (Tabery 2014). This book describes how predisposing genetic factors particular to the individual, interacting with environmental stressors, can be the basis of a general model that can be applied to most categories of mental disorder. I apply these principles to most of the more common conditions that psychiatrists see.

I do not, however, focus on disorders in which the gene-environment model is not quite appropriate, particularly in conditions whose etiology is mainly biological. Thus, I do not discuss autism spectrum disorders, or neurocognitive disorders in which research shows that the environment plays only a minor role. Although schizophrenia is also highly genetic, I discuss research supporting a role for environmental risk factors. I also, much more briefly, describe the weaker evidence for environmental risk in bipolar disorders. I omit many other conditions listed in DSM manuals that are insufficiently researched to determine whether they fit the model.

BEYOND REDUCTIONISM

In recent years, my critique of modern psychiatry has focused on the idea of biological reductionism. The pendulum has swung so far that the effects of psychosocial environment are dismissed, or at best paid lip service. Reductionism in science has had great success but has great limitations. We cannot understand water by reducing it to the properties of hydrogen and oxygen. Complex phenomena have *emergent* properties that cannot be explained by their components (Gillett 2016).

Moreover, the pathways leading to mental disorders are not linear but involve an enormously complex set of interactions. The principle that disorders have multiple causes may seem a truism. Yet contemporary psychiatry honors it "more in the breach than in the observance." Like other disciplines that face complexity, psychiatry has been susceptible to reductionistic theories. We are tempted to reduce cognitive dissonance and to look for simple ways to explain what we observe.

Psychiatry has suffered from what Snow (1958/1993) called the problem of "two cultures." A biomedical mental health culture takes the world view that mental disorders are primarily the result of factors *in-*

side the person. A psychosocial culture takes the world view that mental disorders are primarily the result of factors *outside* the person. Both models tend to be reductionistic, applying unidimensional theories in which one risk factor causes one disorder. The historical background of these models is illuminating. Biological theories dominated psychiatry during the nineteenth century but went into decline in the first half of the twentieth century, largely because few brain abnormalities could be observed and because no effective biological treatments for mental disorders were available. The postwar years were the heyday of psychoanalysis and other psychological therapies. In the latter decades of the twentieth century, however, and even more in the twenty-first century, successful pharmacological treatment came of age, and brain science again came to dominate psychiatric theory. Even so, modern psychiatry still lacks a comprehensive biological theory (Harrington 2019).

These world views suffer from reductionism, even at the biological level. The effects of genes are extremely complicated, and hundreds of them can be involved in a single disorder. Similarly, the role of life events in psychopathology is complex, and one should not assume that single traumatic events cause mental disorders, a complexity that has sometimes led to the use of the term "environome" (Plomin 2018).

The theoretical models that psychiatrists use are not just a matter of intellectual interest. They profoundly affect what these psychiatrists do clinically. If a psychiatrist believes that mental disorders arise from single causes, he or she will tend to treat patients with single methods. In a biomedical model, clinicians search for aberrant neurotransmitter pathways that can be specifically targeted by carefully designed pharmacological agents. In an environmental model, clinicians may search for life events and psychological conflicts or assumptions that can be addressed through psychotherapy. To do justice to the complex causes of psychopathology, we need much more sophisticated explanations of the relationship between risks and disorders (Kendler 2019). Any comprehensive and clinically relevant approach must be multivariate. (Modern statistics reflect this approach, replacing t-tests and chi-squares with regression equations.)

The psychosocial risk factors for psychiatric illness are important, but we must be cautious in attributing pathology of patients to negative events that are common in human life. Because clinicians only see people who became disordered, they tend to develop a distorted view of the relationship between adversity and illness. In biologically vulnerable people, however, negative events have a stronger effect. For example, in PTSD, adverse experiences, unless they activate predispositions, usually cause only short-term, not long-term effects (Yehuda 2002). Many of the associations in the literature between psychosocial risks and mental disorders can be accounted for by predisposed subpopulations.

Thinking interactively helps us avoid assuming simple relationships between causes and effects. Instead, the model encourages us to address complex relationships between many causes and many effects. It also offers a nonreductionistic way of conceptualizing the origins of psychopathology. Unfortunately, reductionism is alive and well. Clinicians of the future need to become more comfortable with complexity. In the long run, the weight of scientific evidence can change the way we think.

THE PURPOSE OF THIS BOOK

My aim is to provide the reader with an intelligible summary of the gene-environment model and to illustrate its application to the understanding of mental disorders. I do not claim to present a new or an original theory. I am hardly the first author to advocate an interactive approach. For those who want to delve further into the details of this subject, I recommend Michael Rutter's (2006) seminal volume *Genes and Behavior*.

In principle, gene-environment interaction theory is in the mainstream of contemporary psychiatry. The idea that diseases arise from interactions between constitution and experience can be traced as far back as the writings of Galen (Monroe and Simons 1991). However, as subdisciplines of psychiatry have become separate and have taken on a narrower vision, interactions have been downplayed. This is particularly true in clinical practice, where ideology too often trumps evidence.

A few words are also needed to explain what this book is *not* about. A great deal of research has been done concerning the precise mechanisms that mediate biological predispositions to mental illness. Yet in spite of all the progress made in recent years, we are still very far from defining how genes act on brain chemistry and connectivity. Therefore, although neuroscience is one of the "hottest" areas of research in psychiatry, this volume only deals with this subject peripherally. One can study genetic influences without knowing exactly how they affect neurotransmitters. Moreover, this is a fast-changing field, in which today's breakthrough often becomes tomorrow's blind alley. In the future, when these issues are better understood, we should be in a position to develop a model fully grounded in neurobiology.

In showing how the model can be usefully applied to a very wide range of psychopathology, I have had to review a very wide literature. Synthesizing this information requires making compromises between the needs of different readers. Specialists may find some sections lacking in detail. However, this book is primarily directed at practicing clinicians. *Its aim is to show how the model should guide evidence-based practice.* Most of the references in this book consist of research reports published in scientific journals, but it is impossible to review a complex literature without picking and choosing. Wherever my conclusions seem controversial, readers should pursue their own inquiries, making use of the extensive reference list provided at the end of this book.

In science, difficult problems are rarely settled by single studies. Only the overall weight of evidence allows firm conclusions. This is why I have referenced many of my conclusions with review articles or books, which are themselves summaries of the research literature. Wherever individual papers shed particular light on questions, I have highlighted them. But as I tell my students, no matter how impressive a research finding is, one needs to wait for a meta-analysis.

THE ARGUMENT OF THE CHAPTERS

Part I: Theory

The first five chapters provide an overview of theories affecting how we study genes, environment, and their interactions and how empirical evidence has shed light on all these issues. They also examine how the theory is transdiagnostic and goes beyond DSM definitions of mental disorders.

Chapter 1: Historical Overview

Over the past 20 years, psychiatry has become much more biological, and contemporary practice is dominated by the use of medication. I highlight studies showing that psychiatrists in practice make much less use of psychotherapy than they did in the past. I argue that the field has moved too radically from one extreme to the other and has failed to integrate nature and nurture, both in theory and practice. Interactive gene-environment models are needed to do justice to the current state of research.

Chapter 2: Genetic Predispositions

Chapter 2 reviews some of the advances in psychiatric genetics over the past two decades. These include such issues as the use of genome-wide association studies and the development of polygenic risk scores. I also review the problems of reductionism in genetics and neuroscience.

Chapter 3: Environmental Stressors

This chapter examines recent research on stress and resilience. Newer ideas that expand the predisposition-stress model, such as differential susceptibility to the environment, are considered. I review a large amount of major longitudinal research that has been carried out in the past two decades, such as the Dunedin Multidisciplinary Health and Development Study, the E-Risk Study, and the Children in the Community Study. These studies show that stressors cannot be understood without considered predispositions, but that environmental events can also make an independent contribution to risk.

Chapter 4: Gene-Environment Interactions

We now have much more evidence, both from behavior genetics and longitudinal research, to shed light on gene-environment interactive mechanisms. I review the various forms of interaction and examine the significance of the contribution of the new discipline of epigenetics.

Chapter 5: Disorders, Diagnoses, and Traits

Chapter 5 addresses some of the unsolved problems in psychiatric diagnosis. Given our current state of knowledge, DSM-5 (American Psychiatric Association 2013) can only be considered as temporarily useful. Categorical diagnoses can be enriched by an understanding of underlying traits. However, dimensional alternatives (the personality disorder model in DSM-5, Section III, and of ICD-11 [World Health Organization 2019], as well as the Hierarchical Taxonomy of Psychopathology [HiTOP; Kotov et al. 2017] system for all mental disorders) seem to be somewhat premature. Along the same lines, I offer commentary on the Research Domain Criteria system (Cuthbert and Insel 2013), which attempts to use neural connectivity to account for psychopathology.

Part II: Mental Disorders

The next eight chapters review evidence on how genes and environment shape the most important mental disorders. I focus on those categories that are frequently seen in practice and that have been extensively researched.

Chapter 6: ADHD and Conduct Disorder

ADHD, often considered to be mainly biological, cannot be understood without considering how heritable temperament interacts with psychosocial adversities and social influences. Conduct disorder arises in childhood, indicating that it is associated with genetic vulnerability, as shown by a large literature.

Chapter 7: Schizophrenia

Psychoses such as schizophrenia are primarily biological in origin. Yet recent evidence shows that they can be triggered by reactions to psychosocial stressors, such as "social defeat" in immigrant populations, and are associated with adverse or traumatic childhood experiences.

Chapter 8: Depressive Disorders

Depressed mood should not be considered just a reflection of chemical imbalances or abnormal neuroconnectivity. Rather, mild to moderate depressions are intimately linked to life events that trigger predispositions, helping to account for the limitations of psychopharmacology in this domain. Chapter 8 also makes brief mention of bipolar disorder, but it does not fit the model, given that research has found it to be highly genetic.

Chapter 9: Anxiety Disorders and Obsessive-Compulsive Disorder

Research on panic disorder and generalized anxiety disorder shows that research on these disorders supports the model. Patients susceptible to anxiety have genetic-temperamental vulnerabilities that often date back to childhood. These tendencies can be amplified by adverse life experiences. OCD is another condition that fits the model. Although we now see this disorder as reflecting a problem in neurocircuitry, it can be triggered by environmental adversities.

Chapter 10: Posttraumatic Stress Disorder

PTSD is not just a response to stressful events but reflects components related to heritable predispositions and environmentally sensitive personality traits. There is also an important social component to the disorder.

Chapter 11: Eating Disorders

The eating disorders, which have greatly increased in prevalence, have been studied intensively over the past two decades. Research provides important support for a model in which heritable predispositions interact with psychological stressors as well as social forces.

Chapter 12: Substance-Related and Addictive Disorders

This group provides an example par excellence of how gene-environment interactions shape psychopathology. A large body of research from the past 20 years is reviewed and shown to support the model.

Chapter 13: Personality Disorders

Personality disorders are my own area of research, and I have a good deal more to say than I did 20 years ago. Gene-environment interactions are essential for understanding these disorders and the traits that underlie them. The development of efficacious specialized therapies for borderline personality disorder demonstrates that even when heritability is fairly strong, an interactive model tends to support specifically designed treatment methods.

Part III: Implications

The final section of the book examines implications of the general model for research and clinical practice.

Chapter 14: Clinical Implications

Psychiatric research has suffered from a failure to study predispositions and stressors in the same populations, effectively preventing investigators from examining their interactions. I provide examples of this problem, drawn from several domains of psychopathology.

Chapter 15: Implications for Prevention and Further Research

Clinical practice, whether psychopharmacological or psychotherapeutic, can benefit from the application of an integrative model. I argue for a model that makes use of both traditions. The chapter also reviews the prospects of prevention for mental disorders, the results of which have been so far discouraging. Here I examine programs for early intervention in mental disorders that begin in youth in which, however aware one is of predispositions and heritability, one can change the course and prognosis of severe mental disorders.

ACKNOWLEDGMENTS

Lise Laporte read the entire manuscript and offered many useful suggestions for improvement. Laura Roberts, Erika Parker, and the American Psychiatric Association Publishing staff offered crucial help and support.

PART I

THEORY

CHAPTER 1

▬ HISTORICAL OVERVIEW

PSYCHIATRY IS a house divided. The division goes back at least a century, and it is rooted in the nature-nurture problem.

Over 60 years ago, in a classic study of psychiatric practice in New Haven, Connecticut, Hollingshead and Redlich (1958) described how psychiatrists fell into two categories: "directive-organic" types who wore white coats and whose therapies consisted mostly of physical treatment, and "analytic-psychological" types who wore jackets and whose treatment methods consisted mainly of talking. Today, clinicians are more eclectic. Even so, psychiatry continues to suffer from an ideological split. Although everyone accepts that both nature and nurture are important, practice is another matter. Some psychiatrists are only interested in symptoms, focus assessment to a DSM-based checklist, and treat patients almost exclusively with medications. Others, now a minority, remain primarily interested in conducting psychotherapy. These differences in practice derive from different models of the causes of mental illness.

For decades, psychiatry has been very different from other branches of medicine. A heavy reliance on psychotherapy made it a subject of suspicion among specialists in other fields. In medical school, students who want to enter psychiatry are still discouraged by comments from faculty, such as "Why would you want to do that? I thought you were smart." The belief that psychiatry should rejoin neurology is an example of this attitude (Insel and Quirion 2005).

Fifty years ago, psychiatry began a slow march into the medical mainstream. It became common for practitioners to believe that most forms of psychopathology derive from biological aberrations and that one should use biological methods to correct them. Psychotherapies went into decline. This change was particularly dramatic in medical schools. Psychoanalysts no longer became department heads. To be successful as an academic psychiatrist, it was better to know about neurons than people.

Ironically, the split between the two cultures of psychiatry continues to bedevil us at the very point when we know more than ever about the causes of mental disorders and have much more effective ways of treating patients. Although psychiatrists still have a long way to go to understand the etiology of mental disorders, their drug treatments are as effective as those of general medicine (Seemüller et al. 2012). Also less well known is the fact that psychotherapy is as effective as medication for common clinical problems such as depression and anxiety (Hunsley et al. 2013). Even if psychiatrists do not always know the causes of the problems they see, they do as well with treatment as most physicians (Leucht et al. 2012).

Yet even today, patients can still receive very different diagnoses and different treatment depending on which kind of clinician they see. Ultimately, the differences between biological and psychosocial models in psychiatry are not based on evidence; rather, they are rooted in *ideology*. Ideas about the etiology of mental disorders mirror larger intellectual questions. The divisions within psychiatry reflect a dichotomy that has been of interest for both philosophers and social scientists: the *nature-nurture problem* (Pinker 2002). This question concerns the extent to which human nature is determined by genes and the extent to which our lives are shaped by environment. Over time, theories taking one side of this controversy or the other have influenced the theory and practice of psychiatry. This chapter undertakes a brief historical overview outlining how these models have influenced clinicians over the past 200 years.

NATURE AND NURTURE IN NINETEENTH-CENTURY PSYCHIATRY

In the course of the nineteenth century, a discipline called "psychiatry" arose out of general medicine and neurology (Shorter 1997). Most practitioners were based in mental hospitals, where the majority of patients had psychotic illnesses. The biological perspective of these early practitioners was therefore entirely natural. In this way, psychiatry in the nineteenth century resembled the ideology of medicine as a whole. Although it was generally acknowledged that the etiology of mental illness was unknown, most clinicians assumed that, as had been the case for many other medical diseases, it was only a matter of time before anatomical or physiological causes of psychopathology would be found.

A number of attempts were made to identify these "constitutional" factors. However, psychiatrists in that century were largely unsuccessful in finding such abnormalities. Inspection of the brain in psychotic patients failed to show pathological changes. (There was one dramatic exception: the identification of general paresis as a tertiary manifestation of syphilitic infection.) In retrospect, we can see that failure was inevitable, given the primitive state of neurobiology at the time (brain imaging was a century away), but the inability of a purely medical model to provide a coherent explanation for psychopathology created an empty niche and led to very different pathways of research. In spite of their overall biological bias, clinicians in the nineteenth century had an interest in the psychological factors of mental illness and practiced early forms of psychotherapy (Ellenberger 1970). From the time of Philippe Pinel and the "moral treatment" of the insane, psychiatrists attempted to apply a psychosocial approach to the treatment of psychotic patients. Some hospitals affiliated with universities, such as the Salpetrière in Paris, and the Burghölzli in Zurich, came to promote psychological models.

The psychiatric paradigms of late nineteenth century are best reflected in the work of the German psychiatrist Emil Kraepelin (1919). In his own time, Kraepelin was the world's most prestigious theorist about mental illness. In recent decades, his ideas have again become influential, leading to the formation of a "neo-Kraepelinian" school (Klerman 1986). Although Kraepelin has been criticized for a supposed lack of humanism, he stood for principles that have remained at the core of his discipline: a focus on the phenomenology of mental illness, a hardheaded empiricism, a refusal to make unnecessary speculations, and a resistance to invoking constructs that cannot be operationalized and measured.

NATURE AND NURTURE IN TWENTIETH-CENTURY PSYCHIATRY

At the turn of the twentieth century, mainstream psychiatry continued to be based on the observation of psychotic patients. This approach was unsatisfactory to a younger generation who wanted to work in innovative and creative ways with a broader population. In this context, the new discipline of psychoanalysis was in a position to attract many clinicians, both medical and nonmedical.

Most practicing analysts did not work in hospitals but treated "neurotic" outpatients in offices and clinics. Psychoanalytic theory not only offered a new way to understand psychopathology but also was a general theory of human psychology (Gellner 1993). The method generated enthusiasm for its therapeutic potential. Psychodynamic ideas also had great impact outside formal analysis on the practice of psychotherapy and on the culture as a whole (Hale 1995).

The institutional structure of psychoanalysis was a factor in the spread of its influence. Freud's decision to create separate pedagogical institutions to promote his ideas encouraged practitioners to make their primary allegiance psychoanalysis rather than psychiatry or medicine. In fact, some of the early analysts were non-M.D. psychologists or teachers.

Between the First and Second World Wars, biological and psychological models contended for the soul of psychiatry. The biological camp could not yet offer adequate treatments for the major psychoses, even though they devised a number of experimental therapies. The only Nobel Prizes in medicine ever awarded to physicians working with psychiatric patients were given to nonpsychiatrists: the Austrian neurologist Wagner-Jauregg, for the malarial treatment of syphilis, and the Portuguese neurosurgeon Moniz, for psychosurgery. (A more recent Nobel Prize awarded to American psychiatrist Eric Kandel was for research on memory.)

After the Second World War, psychiatry was divided into two camps: those who conformed to a medical model and provided organic treatments and psychoanalysts committed to the "talking cure." On the biological side of the divide, electroconvulsive therapy (ECT) was being overused. In the absence of effective medications, ECT—which eventually found its place as an effective treatment for melancholia—was prescribed for all forms of depression (Shorter 1997). Insulin therapy was also a popular method, although it was later discarded when clinical trials failed to demonstrate its effectiveness. Psychosurgery was another psychiatric "fad" that was later almost entirely discredited (Valenstein 1988). Effective biological treatment only became a reality in the 1950s, with the development of antipsychotics and tricyclic antidepressants.

On the psychological side of the divide, psychoanalysis reached the zenith of its influence in the 1950s and 1960s. For a time, training in analysis was almost a "must" qualification to become a chairman of an academic department of psychiatry (Eisenberg 1995). These clinicians were strong on charisma and rhetoric but largely ignorant of research methods. Yet even at its time of greatest dominance, psychoanalysis was itself divided. The movement has always had a tendency to splinter, and many variants of Freud's original model existed. Among the forms of psychotherapy common in the 1960s were "neo-Freudian" variants of psychoanalysis, client-centered therapy, group therapy, behavior therapy, and family therapy. Still, most of these offshoots remained far closer intellectually to psychology than to medicine. As different as these ideas were, most had one important thing in common: they were rooted in theories attributing psychopathology primarily to childhood adversities (Paris 2019).

NATURE AND NURTURE IN TWENTY-FIRST-CENTURY PSYCHIATRY

Today, the profile of theory and practice in psychiatry has greatly changed. As in the previous century, many if not most psychiatrists adhere to biological theories. The fact that we now have pharmacological agents that are effective and have relatively few side effects has had a profound effect on the way clinicians think. When so many disorders are correctable with medication, clinicians are much more tempted to espouse theories reducing psychopathology to "chemical imbalances." The fact that no such imbalances have ever been observed does not seem to discourage those who adopt this ideology.

Today, the psychotherapies have a narrower scope in psychiatry than they once did. One reason for this decline is that psychotherapy was oversold, leading to disappointment and disillusionment (Eisenberg 1986). Although psychotherapeutic methods have been shown by empirical research to be effective for a wide variety of patients (Lambert 2013), they often work more slowly than medications and are much less effective for patients with severe psychopathology. Another issue is that traditional methods of psychotherapy are lengthy, making them expensive and inaccessible. This problem has been at least partially addressed by a move to time-limited brief therapy, which has a strong evidence base.

In contrast, medications for common mental disorders are relatively inexpensive, and prescribing them uses less clinician time. The problem is that only half of all depressed patients have a good response to antidepressants, which have only a narrow advantage over placebo (Kirsch et al. 2008). The idea that antidepressant failure (often called "treatment-resistant depression") can be managed by adding more medications to a "cocktail" may work for a minority of patients, but for most has only slim support from research (see Paris 2010 and Moncrieff 2018 for detailed reviews).

The impact of these ideas has been profound, however. More patients are on psychiatric medication—now about 12% of the U.S. population (Mojtabai 2008; Pratt et al. 2017) than at any other time in history. Another set of effect derives from tendencies to continue prescriptions indefinitely and to put patients on polypharmacy regimes when they do not work, leading to cascades of side effects that are more predictable than good clinical outcomes. As a consultant to family practitioners and to other psychiatrists, I find these problems ubiquitous. Clinicians who believe that depressed patients have chemical imbalances that have little to do with their life circumstances apply this ideology by aggressive prescribing practices. Referrals to psychotherapy may not be made at all or are only considered when depression appears to be stubbornly "treatment resistant." In addition, much continuing medical education is paid for by pharmaceutical companies, and their representatives are frequent visitors to physicians in office practice. "Big Pharma" does not promote medications that have been in use for years (and whose side effects are well known); instead, they promote new medications that tend to be "copycats," with their own side effects, and are much more expensive for consumers.

Meanwhile, psychotherapy remains difficult to access for many patients. It may be insured by managed care plans, but the number of sessions covered is usually lower than what research shows is likely to be effective (Lambert 2013). Moreover, many patients remain uninsured. Thus, the structure of the U.S. mental health system (assuming it deserves to be called a "system") stands in the way of making rational choices between applying a purely biological model or a biopsychosocial approach. Finally, residency training in psychiatry does not always provide adequate preparation for conducting evidence-based psychotherapy. Although few mourn the disappearance of psychoanalytic dominance, programs vary greatly in whether they have teachers who can transmit current knowledge about effective psychosocial treatments.

In theory, combined treatment with medication and psychotherapy remains the most frequently used option for management of common mental disorders, such as depression (Olfson and Marcus 2010), but we do not know the quality of psychological treatment that most patients receive or whether it corresponds to evidence-based standards. Psychiatric models have had an unfortunate history of going from one extreme to another. Decades ago, Grinker (1964) critiqued the unbridled enthusiasm for community psychiatry that characterized his time in a memorable phrase: "psychiatry rushes off in all directions." More than 50 years later, we are still searching for the right direction.

Biological psychiatrists have been insufficiently interested in studying the psychological precipitants of mental disorders. In a witty comment, Lipowski (1989) suggested that whereas the dominance of psychodynamic psychiatry was characterized by "brainlessness," the contemporary biological era is characterized by "mindlessness." There is a real danger that contemporary psychiatrists will lose interest in the person. This would be a tragic outcome of the great achievements of modern biological research. No matter how sophisticated we become in studying the brain, when we stop talking to patients, we lose the soul of our profession. Moreover, we cannot fully understand the origins of mental disorders through their biological correlates. As wise physicians have always known, all illnesses have a unique course, shaped by the events of patients' lives.

At the same time, few psychotherapists have taken the implications of genetic research into account in their work. Most clinicians accept that certain illnesses, particularly schizophrenia and bipolar mood disorder, have a strong genetic component. These cases are rarely referred for psychotherapy, although some evidence has shown that support can make a difference. Unfortunately, some therapists still believe that *other* forms of mental disorder are largely psychological.

As shown in this book, genetic factors are involved in the development of almost *all* forms of pathology, even conditions such as PTSD and personality disorders that have often been considered primarily environmental in origin. Unfortunately, much of the psychotherapy community continues to subscribe to an environmentally reductionistic paradigm, explaining psychic distress as a direct reaction to life events. These clinicians are ignoring the genetic and biological factors underlying even the most common psychological symptoms. The ebb and flow of scientific ideas is not, of course, determined only by fashion. In the long run, theories must stand or fall on the weight of cumulative empirical evidence. Nevertheless, in the short run, there is some relationship between theoretical preferences and cultural values.

Environmental reductionism had its most powerful impact in North America. This may not be a coincidence. Frank and Frank (1991) suggested sociological reasons for the difference between American and European ideas, pointing out that American society deeply values individualism, promoting the belief that individual goals should not be shackled—neither by tradition nor by biological imperatives. The idea that anybody who wants to make something of his or her life can do so with enough persistence is a deeply held value in the culture, often tagged with the phrase "only in America." However, psychiatry in the United States went on to make a 180° turn, prioritizing biology over psychology.

A disparate range of environmentalist theories have been influential in America, including some schools of psychoanalysis, cognitive-behavioral theories, and social models of mental illness. Starting in the 1990s, theories accounting for adult symptoms on the basis of childhood trauma had a large impact on clinicians, as well as on the general public. What all these environmental models have in common is that they attribute the etiology of mental disorders almost entirely to psychological and social factors: traumatic life events, bad families, or a sick society. These ideas are seductive because, however misleading, they contain a grain of truth. There *is* empirical evidence that traumatic life events increase the risk for many forms of psychopathology, that dysfunctional families are more likely to raise children with mental disorders, and that levels of social cohesion affect the prevalence of psychiatric illness (see Chapter 4).

Yet what narrowly environmental models fail to take into account is that associations between risk factors and psychopathology are only statistical correlations that do not prove causality. Moreover, although more people who are exposed to risks will fall ill, most will not. This is because the effects of the environment depend on factors within the person. That interaction is the main theme of this book.

NATURE, NURTURE, AND THE SOCIAL SCIENCES

The nature-nurture debate has also raised sharp controversies in the social sciences. Traditionally, psychology, sociology, and anthropology have all emphasized environmental influences on individual differences. Steven Pinker (2002) described a "standard social science model" as a version of seventeenth-century philosopher John Locke's concept that children are a "blank slate" on which the environment writes a script.

The resistance of the social sciences to integrating biology has been fierce and often bitter. Sociobiology, as described by E.O. Wilson (1975), is a theory that explains universal human behavioral patterns in terms of natural selection, but Wilson was attacked by Marxist biologists for these ideas (Segerstråle 2000). Although Wilson is a noted Harvard entomologist and a lifelong liberal Democrat, he had to endure a physical attack at a conference when an opponent poured ice water on him. When he came to speak in my own city of Montreal in the 1970s, a sociology professor, who probably had not read anything Wilson had written, asked me if I wanted to help a protest against the lecture. (Yes, even then, speakers could be shouted down by "activists.")

Evolutionary psychology is a closely related discipline (Buss 2019). It has endured similar attacks, probably because it challenged a postwar consensus that environment explains everything, resisting any application of evolution and genetics to the social sciences.

What was all this drama about? It comes down to politics. If you believe in Marxism or other Utopian ideas, then you must believe that there is nothing to the concept of human nature and that humans are a blank slate. It follows that a just society can be built through hard work and idealism. If, on the other hand, you are conservative, you are likely to believe that there are limits to the reform of society, based on a delicate balance between selfishness and cooperation. The libertarian social commentator Thomas Sowell (2010) described these points of views as "unconstrained" vs. "constrained" visions of the human condition. Pinker (2002) reformulated these points of view as a "utopian vision" vs. a "tragic vision." Later, Pinker (2018) welcomed the progress that has been made in the quality of human life since the Enlightenment, but does not believe in perfection. These views continue to meet resistance from leftist thinkers.

Although I support a tragic vision of human nature, that does not mean treating patients is not useful or important. What it does mean is that one should not have utopian goals, either by correcting errors in human biology or by teaching people how to live better.

Another domain in the social sciences in which nature and nurture clash is the scientific study of human intelligence. The evidence is clear that IQ is heritable at the same level as other traits (Plomin 2018). Yet some have believed that these findings are artificial and even have racist implications (Lewontin et al. 1984). Scarr (1991) discussed why the genetic factors in intelligence and personality are resisted or dismissed by so many people and asked, "Why the resistance to the idea that parents transmit genes to their children, with the consequence that their children resemble them to a modest extent? Because behavioral scientists understand genetic transmission to mean that nothing can be done to change the unfortunate lot of people who inherit bad genes" (p. 385). The contrary is true. As opportunities become more equal, individual differences tend to stand out more dramatically. As Scarr (1991) went on to point out, "egalitarian provisions *raise* the heritability of personal and intellectual characteristics in Western populations" (p. 386). That is why intelligence is less heritable in African Americans, where poverty interferes with education (Plomin 2018).

NATURE, NURTURE, AND MODERN MEDICINE

Although the genetic lottery may not be fair, an understanding of how it affects individuals can help us take a more humane view of mental illness.

When we recognize that patients have inherent areas of vulnerability, we need hold neither them nor those in their immediate environment entirely responsible for their problems. When we treat patients, we can provide them with whatever forms of treatment have been shown to be effective, without being judgmental. Thus, acknowledging the genetic factors in mental disorders need not lead to determinism or despair. Instead, it can be the basis of a higher form of humanism.

The triumph of modern medicine means that we usually recover from periods of acute illness and live much longer. As a result, the focus of medical research and care has shifted to chronic diseases. This makes it much closer to psychiatry. Historically, medical genetics concerned relatively rare conditions with classical Mendelian inheritance. However, chronic illnesses, like mental disorders, arise from complex genetic patterns and multiple risks from the environment.

A large body of evidence supports the principle that the genetic susceptibility to common chronic illnesses such as coronary artery disease, essential hypertension, or diabetes mellitus involves polygenic mechanisms of inheritance, amplified by environmental risks (Kendler 1995). As each genetic factor interacts with other genes, overall liability can cross a threshold and determine whether overt disease develops, as well as the severity of illness. One example is the "two-hit model" of carcinogenesis, in which pathology depends both on biology (the mutation of genes that stimulate cell proliferation and the deactivation of tumor suppression genes) and environmental mechanisms (Knudson 1996). For example, people with a heritable predisposition to lung cancer are much more likely to develop the disease if they also smoke. The same idea has been applied by to schizophrenia (Maynard et al. 2001). The theory is that a heritable (and/or intrauterine) risk factor disrupts brain development but only causes disease when a second hit occurs in adolescence or young adulthood.

Genetic susceptibility is a *necessary* condition for the development of most chronic medical illnesses and can determine which type of illness an individual can develop. It is not, however, a *sufficient* condition for most diseases, which will only become clinically apparent when environmental factors increase liability. These theories may also explain why the same illness in different individuals can have a different onset and course. When genetic factors are stronger, illness often tends to develop at an earlier age. When diseases have an early onset, there has not been sufficient time for environmental risks to accumulate and provoke the onset. They are therefore more likely to be associated with a stronger genetic loading (Childs and Scriver 1986). Conversely, a disease that develops later in life is more likely to be influenced by relatively weaker genetic factors but by stronger environmental factors: the older the person is, the longer the time available for environment stressors to exert their cumulative effects. Behavioral genetics shows that death occurring *before* the age of 60 years depends strongly on inheritance, whereas death *after* age 60 is more strongly related to environmental factors (Sørensen et al. 1988).

As a researcher in cardiac disease once summarized the model: "Most major chronic diseases probably result from the accumulation of environmental factors over time in genetically susceptible persons" (Williams 1988, p. 770). Natural selection leads organisms to evolve mechanisms of resilience against disease so that only the cumulative effects of multiple environmental insults will overwhelm these defenses. These models of disease apply well to mental disorders. In psychiatry, the nature-nurture debate can only be resolved through recognition of interaction between genes, the cumulative effects of environmental adversity and the effects of risk factors on vulnerable individuals. This principle needs to be confirmed through careful examination of empirical evidence. The rest of this book is devoted to that task.

CHAPTER 2

▬ GENETIC PREDISPOSITIONS

NATURAL SELECTION is the key to biology. All organisms are programmed to survive and reproduce. A master plan coded in the genes shapes all phenotypic traits, including anatomical structures, physiological functioning, and behavior. These programs are laid down in two types of genes: a smaller number that code for the synthesis of specific proteins and a larger number that regulate the development of fertilized eggs into complex organisms.

Although almost all human characteristics are guided by the genome, there is no simple correspondence between genotypes and phenotypes. As pointed out by Pinker (2007), "a single gene rarely specifies some identifiable part of an organism. Instead it specifies the release of a protein at specific times in development, an ingredient of an unfathomably complex recipe, usually in having some effect in molding a suite of parts that are affected by other genes" (pp. 321–322). Thus, decoding the human genome still left us a long way from being able to describe how changes at the level of a genetic code to thoughts, emotions, and behavior. As Pinker (2007) explains:

> the relationship between particular genes and particular psychological traits is doubly indirect. First, a single gene does not build a single brain module; the brain is a delicately layered soufflé in which each gene product is an ingredient with a complex effect on many properties of many circuits. Second, most of the traits which capture our attention emerge out of unique combinations of kinks in many different modules. (p. 328)

Traits are not, therefore, controlled by heredity like a puppet on a genetic string. Genes code for proteins, not behaviors. Thus, there is no such thing as a gene "for shyness," a gene "for criminality," or a gene "for depression." Rather, each of these psychological traits is influenced by interactions between many gene loci, and between genes and the environment.

The relationship between behavioral traits and phenotypes is particularly complex and knotty (Rutter 2006). We often observe genetic heterogeneity, in which the same outcome can emerge from different combinations of genes. In addition, the same combination of genes can lead to different outcomes because the expression of genes can be entirely different under different environmental conditions.

Many genes are inoperative unless "turned on" by the environment, which is the basis of *epigenetics*—the study of how life experience affects genetic activity (Ward 2018). This is one of the reasons why it is not possible to make precise predictions about phenotypes in any individual. Also, the importance of epigenetics is shown by the fact that identical twins are not totally identical (Ward 2018). Yet although epigenetics is currently a "hot" subject in research, its precise role in shaping behavioral differences is not firmly established (Gorman 2018). Thus, much of the research on this mechanism has been on rodents, and it is not known how applicable these findings are to our own species. In contrast, behavioral genetics has already proven itself to be one of the most powerful tools for measuring how genes affect behavior.

EXPLAINING INDIVIDUAL DIFFERENCES

Human beings differ greatly one from another. They look different, have different intellectual capacities, develop different personality traits, and develop different diseases. Moreover, individual differences in personality traits are associated with differential vulnerabilities to mental disorders (Plomin et al. 2013). Any comprehensive theory of psychopathology must take these variations into account. Individual differences can result from nature or nurture, but their interactions provide the most adequate explanation of why individuals differ from each other.

With the exception of monozygotic twins, none of us have precisely the same genes. (Even in identical twins, epigenetic differences accumulate over the lifespan.) Genetic differences impose limits on the forms environmentally induced expressions of traits can take, but these individual differences can be either amplified or suppressed by the environment. A good example is the relationship between personality traits and personality disorders (see Chapter 13). Each personality type is potentially adaptive, and trait differences need not necessarily be pathological (Beck et al. 2014; Belsky and Pluess 2009; Boyce 2019). Some traits, when amplified to dysfunctional levels, can lead to significant psychopathology, but dysfunction becomes more likely when traits are not buffered by interactions with other, more adaptive traits or when environmental factors lead to amplification.

Consider, for example, extraversion-introversion, a basic dimension of personality that varies normally in the population (Widiger and Costa 2013). These traits can sometimes be problematical, either because they are unusually intense by nature or because environmental factors related to nurture lead to their amplification. Within a normal range, extraverts are charming and attractive people. However, at a certain point, it can be dysfunctional to be excessively extraverted, if you are excessively dependent on the responses of others. Similarly, introversion is normally functional and is associated with useful self-sufficiency. Yet amplification of introverted traits can lead to avoidance and social isolation. Another example of the complexity of traits under genetic influence is that the environment can suppress genetic differences. As discussed in Chapter 1, intelligence is an example. Thus, although strong evidence has been found for the heritability of intellectual capacities, differences are much less common in socially disadvantaged populations, "flattening out" genetic effects.

Another reason for complexity is that many genes associated with illness remain in the population because, by themselves, they have no pathogenic consequences. These variations in penetrance and expressivity are related to environmental factors. Thus, the environment is a major determinant of whether a predisposition remains latent or leads to overt illness. For each predisposed individual who falls ill, many others develop no illness at all or only develop subclinical symptoms. Consider adult-onset diabetes mellitus type 2. The genes that constitute this predisposition are widely distributed but only lead to disease when the food supply makes obesity possible (Gross et al. 2004). In the environments in which humanity evolved, the diabetic gene might actually have protected its carriers from starvation by allowing for a more rapid breakdown of fat stores. In our present environment of abundance, the same genes can cause disease. This relationship also explains why many patients with diabetes can be treated simply by restricting their diet.

HERITABILITY AND CHRONIC DISEASE

Historically, medical genetics focused on relatively rare conditions with a classical Mendelian inheritance. Now the main direction of research involves identifying multiple genetic interactions associated with diseases based on complex traits.

The genetic susceptibility to common chronic diseases usually involves polygenic mechanisms of inheritance (Lvovs et al. 2012). Some of the most important of these illnesses are coronary artery disease, essential hypertension, diabetes mellitus, and schizophrenia. When phenotypes depend on interactions between multiple loci, some genes will increase the risk for illness while others will reduce the risk. As each genetic factor interacts with environmental factors, overall liability can cross a threshold and determine whether overt disease develops, as well as the severity of illness.

Genetic susceptibility is therefore a *necessary* condition for the development of most chronic diseases and also determines which type of illness the individual is likely to develop. It is not, however, a *sufficient* condition for most diseases, which only become clinically apparent when environmental factors trigger symptoms. As a researcher in cardiac disease once remarked: "Most major chronic diseases probably result from the accumulation of environmental factors over time in genetically susceptible persons" (Williams 1988, p. 769).

Just as predispositions are polygenic, stressors tend to be polyenvironmental. Natural selection leads organisms to evolve mechanisms of resilience against disease so that only the cumulative effects of multiple environmental insults can overwhelm these defenses. This is why the cumulative effect of psychosocial adversities is more predictive of psychopathology than any single life event, and a large literature shows that mental disorders and psychosocial stressors reduce life expectancy.

Chronic diseases are heterogeneous in etiology. The same illness in different individuals can reflect different degrees of genetic and environmental influence. When genetic factors are stronger, illness tends to develop at an earlier age. When diseases have an early onset, environmental risks have not had time to accumulate; therefore, these diseases are more likely to be associated with stronger genetic loading. Conversely, a disease that develops later in life is more likely to be influenced by relatively weaker genetic factors but by stronger environmental factors. The older a person is, the more time has been available for environmental stressors to exert cumulative effects. Moreover, diseases that begin in old age may not affect the capacity for reproduction and are therefore less likely to be eliminated by natural selection.

When we apply for life insurance, the company probes our medical status through a series of investigations. The insurer tends to focus on a few basic issues: whether one can pass a physical examination and whether common markers of vulnerability to illness, such as glucose levels and blood pressure, are within normal limits. Before being tested, one is required to answer a list of questions on an insurance form. Perhaps the most important item on the questionnaire concerns the longevity of our parents. From large actuarial databanks on survival, insurers know that, on average, they can make more money on those of us who have long-lived parents, and they are more likely to lose money on those of us whose parents had the misfortune to die young. As noted in Chapter 1, premature death is strongly influenced by genetic factors, given that diseases that affect people only after reproduction are not subject to natural selection (Sørensen et al. 1988).

Yet it has not always been true that a short life span depends on genetic vulnerability. Today, most people live out an extended life span and die of diseases of old age, such as myocardial infarction, stroke, or cancer. Yet until quite recently, infectious diseases were the major cause of premature death. In spite of the AIDS epidemic, the mortality among young people from infection has never been lower than it is today. Even so, genetic factors also play some role in liability to infectious diseases by influencing the strength of immunity (Childs et al. 1992). For example, heredity is one factor that predicts whether one is likely to develop tuberculosis (Rumyantsev 1992). About 10% of the North American population have a genetic resistance to developing HIV infection (Dean et al. 1996). However, the heritable factors in infectious diseases are generally weaker than in chronic diseases.

Research has aimed to describe these hereditary predispositions. This has raised the hope that one day we will receive a gene profile telling us which diseases we are most prone to develop. However, progress in this area has not been rapid. People should be cautious about relying on commercial products that test DNA and report on risk levels that have a very weak statistical relationship to any outcome. In principle, we could use such information to change habits, by avoiding specific environmental stressors. In practice, at our present state of knowledge, these procedures have little value.

Genetics has traditionally been concerned only with biological factors, whereas epidemiology has focused on environmental factors in disease. In contrast, genetic epidemiology has the goal of combining both in a single discipline, elucidating the mechanisms by which environmental factors determine pathways from predispositions to overt pathology (Teare 2011). This research program conducts studies in large populations to examine the interactions of genes and environment in the etiology of human disease. However, these relationships are not simple, and outcome reflects a complex combination of genetic factors.

EVOLUTION AND HUMAN DISEASE

Natural selection is a mechanism that maximizes fitness to the environment. What evolutionary theory means by *fitness* is the extent to which genes affect the likelihood that organisms successfully reproduce. This leads to a question: given that genes are a product of natural selection, why do pathogenic genetic variants remain in the population? This question about why humans remain prone to disease is a central concern for *evolutionary psychiatry* (Brune 2015; Nesse 2019; Nesse and Williams 1994).

Two lines of inference help account for this paradox. First, natural selection acts only on those characteristics that influence reproductive capacity. Genes that increase the likelihood of developing diseases prior to or during the reproductive years tend to be selected out of the population. At the same time, genes that lead to disease only later in life can remain in the gene pool, because genes that express themselves only *after* reproduction are immune to natural selection. A well-known example of this principle is Huntington's disease (Walker 2007). This illness is caused by a dominant gene associated with the presence of an abnormal genetic sequence termed *trinucleotide repeats*. Once the disease begins, usually in middle age, it is incurable and eventually fatal. Yet because the gene has no effect in the reproductive years, it is transmitted to offspring and remains in the population.

The second reason organisms remain vulnerable to disease is that body plans developed by evolution are not perfect (Nesse 2019). There is always a trade-off between the cost and benefit of any adaptation. Every species has inborn protective mechanisms against disease. However, a balance in natural selection occurs between the effectiveness of a protection and its energy cost to the organism. Most aspects of organismic design represent compromises between these conflicting forces. For example, the large and complex human brain brings many selective advantages but is also associated with significant costs, such as high levels of morbidity during childbirth. Moreover, some genetic effects are accidents of history, "pleiomorphic" traits that were selected for another purpose but lead to unanticipated consequences. The process of aging itself might be due to both of these processes: accumulated genetic effects acting later in the life cycle and intrinsic design flaws in the organism. These factors may explain why senescence is biologically inevitable (Nesse and Williams 1994).

Genetically determined diseases frequently affect young people. This is most particularly the case in psychiatry. To understand why, we can review some mechanisms of genetic transmission. The gene pool in any population is subject to a constant process of mutation. Most of these mutations reduce fitness and are quickly selected out of the population, but the rare mutations that increase fitness fire the engine of evolution. Genetic variations in any trait can either be positive, negative, or neutral depending on environmental conditions. For example, genes increasing rates of fat storage are adaptive under conditions of famine but are maladaptive when food is abundant (Nesse 2019). Thus, characteristics that evolved for adaptation in one environment can be maladaptive in a different environment.

In classic Mendelian heredity, traits are essentially either "on" or "off." However, this simple dichotomy is the exception, not the rule. For single genes, in some cases of recessive inheritance, heterozygotes can still be affected less severely by an abnormal trait. In some diseases there may even be a selective advantage to heterozygosity, with the result that the genes are more likely to remain in the population. This phenomenon is termed *balanced polymorphism*. This mechanism is exemplified by sickle cell anemia. Although this disease is severe and life-threatening, the gene for the trait remains common in African populations. The reason is that this heterozygosity, by shaping the red blood cells in a sickle shape, makes it more difficult for a parasite to survive. This protects carriers against malaria, which is highly endemic in Africa. However, in the malaria-free North American environment, heterozygosity has no advantage, and massive sickling in homozygous individuals leads to serious illness.

These classical examples of genetic risk still depend on Mendelian transmission. Yet with few exceptions, mental disorders have a complex heritability that involves hundreds or thousands of genes. These complex pathways to genetic vulnerability can be studied in twin samples.

USING TWIN SAMPLES TO MEASURE HERITABILITY

Heritability is a quantitative estimate of the extent to which any trait is inherited. The measurement of heritability has a long and distinguished history in medical research. Studies can be conducted in either community or clinical samples, but findings drawn from population-based research are more broadly generalizable whereas clinical samples are usually biased in one way or another.

Family history is a classical method of looking for evidence of heritability. This approach is unable to separate the effects of genes and environment. Nonetheless, whenever family history studies have suggested that disorders have a genetic component, twin or adoption studies have confirmed this conclusion (Plomin 2018). Thus, the presence of a positive family history of any disorder can be regarded as at least presumptive of genetic risk.

The best way to estimate heritability of any trait is *behavior genetics*. The method uses twin samples, with a heritability coefficient calculated from differences in concordance between monozygotic and dizygotic twins. These differences can be translated into a quantitative measure of heritability, usually expressed as a percentage. A finer-grained procedure is called *model fitting*, in which one tests how well several different models (genetic, environmental, or mixed genetic-environmental) account for these differences. Computer modeling can then separate out two types of genetic effects, termed *additive* and *nonadditive*. Additive effects occur when a number of genetic factors add more or less equal increments to the phenotype, whereas nonadditive effects point to the presence of a major Mendelian gene.

There are three caveats to keep in mind about the interpretation of twin studies. First, it is misleading to think that heritability, expressed as a percentage, reflects the precise strength of genetic influence in any single person. Rather, it measures to what extent individual differences in a trait *within a population* can be accounted for by genes. Thus, heritability estimates do not apply to individuals, in whom genes or environment can have greater or lesser contributions to outcome, but to group averages. In other words, different individuals can have greater or lesser genetic contributions to the same trait. Second, the percentage of variance attributable to heredity depends on the population under study. Because the ultimate effects of genes depend on interactions with the environment, the same trait can have different degrees of heritability in different socioeconomic groups or in different societies.

A third issue concerns the equal environments assumption. If monozygotic twins have a more similar environment than dizygotic twins, heritability is being overestimated by current methods. This argument has gone on for several decades. A meta-analysis of 50 years of research (Polderman et al. 2015) supported the equal environments assumption. Thus, a wide body of data continues to show that there are only minor differences in the rearing of identical and fraternal twins by parents, although the exact percentages may be somewhat elevated (Uher and Zwicker 2017), but that does not challenge the model as a whole. Interestingly, twins raised apart are *more* similar than those raised together, probably because twins who are raised together often try to minimize their differences and come to resemble each other more as they grow older (Plomin et al. 2013).

Other questions that have been raised about the validity of twin studies are of less concern (Plomin 2018). For example, no unique characteristics have been found in twins that are not found in non-twins. Some of the criticism has been tendentious, given that there are at least as many problems in interpreting studies of nongenetic factors in disease. Some still want to discount genetics on the mistaken grounds that genes are always deterministic.

One of the most interesting applications of twin methodology is that it can also be used to estimate the *environmental* factors affecting human traits (Knopik et al. 2017). In addition to determining the percentage of genetic influence on individual differences for any trait, we can also calculate the influence of two types of environmental factors. The first type depends on similarities between individuals related to living in the same family and social setting and is called the *shared environment*. The second type is the *unshared environment*, which reflects differences in experiences within the same family, differential niches in the family, or the effects of life experiences outside the family. The surprise has been that, contrary to what past theorists would have predicted, most of the environmental variance affecting psychopathology (as well as personality and intelligence) is unshared. This is one of the most important findings on the history of human sciences. It contradicts the simplistic assumption that families and societies breed mental illness.

The heritability of personality (generally about 40%–50%) has an importance all its own. Personality traits are important predisposing factors for major psychiatric illnesses (Krueger and Tackett 2003). once compared personality to an immune system, processing environmental stimuli of all kinds. Even the environmental factors in behavior are partly a function of the genes. Thus, genetically shaped traits shape a child's intellectual environment, so that intelligent children gravitate toward experiences that facilitate intellectual development (Scarr and McCartney 1983). In several ways, therefore, genes influence the overall quality of life experience.

ADOPTION STUDIES

Studies of adopted children are useful for addressing the problem of separating genetic and environmental factors in disease. If adoptees are more similar to their biological parents than to their adoptive parents, this provides very strong evidence indeed for heritability of a trait. Studies of both intelligence and personality traits show similarities on many traits between adopted children and their biological parents and only weak relationships to the adoptive parents (Knopik et al. 2017). Adoption studies are few, but wherever they have been carried out on mental disorders, they yield findings that parallel those of twin studies.

Most criticisms of the adoption method can be readily dismissed (Knopik et al. 2017). Thus, there is no evidence that the process used to place them for adoption has an effect on behavior or that the psychological effects of adoption itself lead to major pathogenic effects. These objections can hardly explain data showing that biological children of a schizophrenic mother are more likely to develop schizophrenia, even when they grow up in normal adoptive families.

Studies of twins separated at birth combine the advantages of both the twin and adoption methods. This is a powerful way to measure heritability, but cases are understandably few. However, a large-scale project conducted at the University of Minnesota collected subjects from all over the United States. The results were widely reported in the media, often punctuated by picturesque anecdotes exemplifying surprising similarities between separated twins. The quantitative findings of this study strongly supported earlier research showing dramatic similarities in both intelligence and personality between twins reared apart (Tellegen et al. 1988).

IMPLICATIONS OF BEHAVIORAL GENETICS FOR PSYCHIATRY

Behavioral genetics has in some ways overthrown some of the most favored past theories in developmental psychology. reviewed the most replicated findings in the field, of which the most important is that all psychological traits show significant and substantial genetic influence. For almost any trait one can think of, about half the population variance will be genetic, and the level of heritable influence usually lies between 40% and 50% (Knopik et al. 2017). The same roughly 50/50 split applies to most of the mental disorders listed in DSM-5 (American Psychiatric Association 2013; Kendler and Prescott 2006). In almost every case, the environmental variance is unshared.

In severe mental disorders, the heritable portion of the variance is higher. Thus, the heritability of schizophrenia has been estimated at 81% (Sullivan et al. 2003) and the heritability of bipolar disorder has been estimated at 85% (McGuffin et al. 2003). These large percentages initially led researchers to look for either single Mendelian genes or a small group of interacting genes, but this search did not prove fruitful.

THE GREAT DISAPPOINTMENT

With the decipherment of the human genome in 2003, many researchers hoped that genes could be mapped sufficiently to explain vulnerability to mental disorders. To this end, the genome has been scanned in great detail. Yet the result of 20 years of research has been a great disappointment. Most attempts to locate genes that can influence psychopathology on specific chromosomes have failed. It turns out that individual genes or a small group of genes do not account for the level of genetic influence found in twin studies. This problem has been called the "missing heritability" (Manolio et al. 2009). These failures led to great disappointment. We have since learned that genes interact with each other and that thousands, each common but with small effects, could be related to every mental disorder.

Another complication is that the majority of sites on the genome do not make proteins but regulate the activity of genes. As shown by a genetic mega-project, the ENCODE consortium found that noncoding DNA is not "junk," as some had suggested, but is biologically active (Parrington 2015). These sites seem to function much like a dimmer switch (Carey 2015). As with most stories in science, things turn out to be more complicated that we expect.

All this research shows that mental disorders have a polygenic, non-Mendelian mechanism involving many gene loci that are each insufficient to cause illness but that increase the risk when in concert. This has been called "complex inheritance." Although many experts expected to find major genes affecting conditions such as schizophrenia and bipolar disorder, these associations are either absent or account for a very small percentage of the variance. Psychiatrists dream of being in a position to identify individual predispositions to disease before illnesses actually develop. Achieving this goal will not be easy. The human genome includes about 30 billion base pairs, with about 20,000 genes. Finding any one gene, or several genes, strongly related to a disease involves searching for multiple needles in multiple haystacks.

Several methods have been used (McGuffin et al. 2004). *Genetic association* involves gathering data showing that changes at gene loci are associated with specific diseases. *Genetic linkage* involves finding precise chromosomal locations of genes associated with disease or with predispositions to disease. Linkage analysis depends on the possibility that a trait under study is on the same chromosome and lies close to the locus of a known genetic marker. A related approach is the *sibling-pair method* (Poznik et al. 2006). Siblings would ordinarily be expected to share genes about half the time, but if two siblings are both affected by the same illness, and if the sharing of a marker is above the chance rate, then this region of the chromosome may contain a gene associated with susceptibility to the disease under study.

None of these methods has led to well-replicated findings linking major mental disorders to gene loci. We have come to realize that mental illness is associated with an even more highly complex inheritance. Moreover, only a few genes have been specifically associated with a major mental disorder, but they account for very little. One example is the relationship between a q22 deletion and schizophrenia (Tang et al. 2017); this deletion is found in only a small minority of patients with schizophrenia and is probably only one of a very large number of pathways to psychosis.

Over the last decade, a very large number of studies using either genetic association methods or genetic linkages have been conducted. By and large, many studies have failed to find alleles that account for a large percentage of the variance (and we do not know how many ended up in the file drawer due to the difficulty of publishing negative findings). Moreover, when genetic relationships are identified, they have a way of disappearing entirely when replications are conducted. This is part of a more general problem in medical and psychological sciences called the *replication crisis* (Ioannidis 2005). Because of small samples and random findings, initial studies tend to show more of an effect than do attempts at replication. The lesson is that no matter how widely quoted a paper is (even if it is promoted in the media), one should never believe any finding unless it is replicated in several different populations and preferably subject to meta-analysis.

Unfortunately, journals tend to prefer striking results that fail to replicate, and it can take years to find out that they are not reliable. The replicability problem has affected many areas of psychiatry, including pharmacological trials and imaging studies, and is a serious problem for psychiatric genetics.

GENOME-WIDE ASSOCIATION STUDIES

Researchers therefore developed a method for scanning the entire genome: the *genome-wide association study* (GWAS) (Bush and Moore 2012). It is favored over past methods that turned out to be unfruitful. A GWAS allows us to study *all* polymorphisms associated with any well-defined disease (Bush and Moore 2012). Again, hopes were high, but the results have been a shocker. They show that diseases with a complex inheritance reflect small effects from *hundreds* or *thousands* of genes (Arribas-Ayllon et al. 2019). That is what we find in almost all major mental disorders.

Some of this negative research has been published as though it were positive, particularly of any genes have a statistically significant relationship to the disorder. However, these results only tell us whether any sites on the genome are associated more often in those affected than in control subjects. The amount of variance accounted for by any one or all of these polymorphisms is almost always small (often around 1%).

There is a way of attempting to get around this problem. One can compute a *polygenic risk score* (PRS), which provides a weighted estimate of how much of the outcome is accounted for by the genome as a whole. Yet these scores still fail to account for much about the genetic factors behind most forms of mental disorder. A PRS still only predicts, at best, about 10% of the variance, even in highly genetic outcomes such as first-episode psychosis (Vassos et al. 2017). Moreover, genetic effects run across disorders and are not generally specific to categories of illness (Cross-Disorder Group of the Psychiatric Genomics Consortium 2019).

It is also notable that most of the sites identified by GWASs do not code for proteins but are involved in gene regulation. These mechanisms remain poorly understood. Uher and Zwicker (2017) reviewed this literature and noted that when we apply polygenic risk scores to data from GWASs,

> analyses consistently show that the prediction of mental illness improves by including more weakly associated genetic variants, suggesting that many thousands of genetic variants are involved in shaping the risk for most mental disorders. These involve both common single nucleotide polymorphisms and rare structural variants, such as deletions and insertions of stretches of DNA. Another consistent finding is that most common and rare genetic variants are nonspecifically associated with a range of mental disorders. (p. 121)

IMPLICATIONS OF GENETIC RESEARCH FOR PSYCHIATRY

Clearly, the mind-boggling complexity of the genome is greater than most of us thought. Genetic effects on mental illness will take many decades to unravel. It is also possible that we are hamstrung by the use of invalid diagnostic categories.

Another striking finding from GWAS research is that genetic risk factors are far from specific to categories of mental disorder, at least as defined by DSM-5. Many of the same genes are associated with risk for depression, bipolar disorder, and schizophrenia (Rasic et al. 2014). This raises the question of whether the classical theory of Kraepelin separating schizophrenia and bipolar disorder is correct. Evidently, these disorders seriously overlap, and what the PRS seems to measure is not genes for either one but for psychosis itself. Thus, although it was once hoped that DSM-defined disorders would be highly correlated with biological markers, it is now clear that they are not. This is a further disappointment and a reason for disillusionment with the validity of DSM itself.

Research on biological markers for disease is one of the major thrusts of contemporary medical research. When a biological marker is consistently associated with a disorder, it suggests the existence of underlying genetic factors. However, biological markers may only reflect the secondary effects of illness and need not always have etiological significance. To make this distinction, we need to know whether the marker was there before the illness developed or is a result of a pathological process initiated by the disorder. Psychiatrists would eventually like to be able to make diagnoses much in the same way as internists, confirming their clinical impressions by carrying out laboratory tests. Thus far, the search for markers specific to mental disorders has been frustrating. Many of the most promising measures have turned out to have a nonspecific relationship to psychopathology.

There are two possible explanations for the lack of a definite relationship between neurochemical or neurophysiological findings and specific mental disorders. First and foremost, even after the "decade of the brain," we still know little about how this organ actually works. Present technology has become sophisticated and impressive, particularly imaging techniques that allow us to study the brain in vivo, but succeeding generations may view these efforts as primitive. Although neuroscience has greatly advanced our understanding of the normal brain, it has done much less for understanding the abnormal. Second, biological markers are usually more related to the traits than underlie disease rather than to overt disorders. In other words, diseases do not constitute phenotypes; instead, we are looking for *endophenotypes*, separating behavioral symptoms into more stable processes that have a genetic connection. However, because illnesses are also dependent on environmental factors, disorder-specific biological markers have not been found.

In light of the lack of specificity of genes or biomarkers to disorders, some researchers have been interested in *transdiagnostic* measures. One of these is the *psychopathology factor*, or *p factor*, a broad measure of illness related to brain changes in a wide range of disorders (Elliott et al. 2018). Yet in spite of all these advances, we have a very long way to go. It has often been said that breakthroughs are "around the corner." Although every few years experts claim that one must only wait for a few more years to pass before research in this area comes to fruition, progress remains around the corner.

Some enthusiasts believe otherwise. In the view of Nobel Prize winner Eric Kandel (2018), we are on the brink of solving the problem. A review in *Science* was also very optimistic, suggesting: "The next few years will undoubtedly see a radical transformation of our understanding of the biological origins of all neuropsychiatric disorders" (Geschwind and Flint 2015, p. 1493). In my view, these hopes are not likely to be fulfilled any time soon. The causes of mental illness are not a project for a few years or a few decades but for a century. We need to be patient and not believe in false promises.

CHAPTER 3

ENVIRONMENTAL STRESSORS

THINKING ABOUT ENVIRONMENTAL RISK

It is difficult to think about environmental risk outside a genetic context, but if there is no Mendelian mechanism, genes do not, as many once believed, determine a life course. Rather, they have a statistical relationship to psychopathology and functioning. Heritable factors can raise risk, but there are few predictable relationships between the genome and human behavior.

Much the same can be said about the environment. Its relation to psychopathology and functioning is also statistical. If risk is raised to a certain level, one can speak of a limited degree of causality, but these risks will usually only affect a minority of those who are exposed to them. One should be aware that even when relationships between risk and outcome are statistically significant in a research study, that does not make them predictive. In clinical practice, we constantly see people who have been exposed to known risks but are unaffected.

There is a dose-response effect for adverse life events. In a community study, Rutter (1989) found that adding up a variety of risk factors to make a score did a better job of predicting the appearance of symptoms in children than did any life event alone. The implication is that no single stressor is determinative, whereas the cumulative effect of multiple stressors over time has some predictive value (Rutter 1987a). Rutter's research, as well as that of numerous others, also demonstrates the role of resilience in development. The sources of resilience are complex

31

(Rutter 2013). To some extent, it reflects the influence of positive traits—heritable characteristics that aid access to more positive experiences and help protect people against mental disorders. Resilience reflects the influence of positive and helpful people in the environment who can buffer the effects of negative and unhelpful people. Finally, resilience may also reflect good luck, which can yield turning points in development.

To summarize, predisposing genetic factors are necessary but usually not sufficient conditions for the development of mental disorders. Environmental stressors are also rarely sufficient, but the environment determines whether predispositions cross a threshold of liability and develop into diagnosable disorders. In this context, it is clear why empirical research does not support the primacy of early childhood experience. Adverse experiences in life at any stage need not lead to mental disorders. The impact of stressors is mediated by individual characteristics, expressed through personality traits. The effects are cumulative, with multiple negative events having more long-term effects than single events. In both childhood and adulthood, resilience is the rule. Thus, some individuals require high levels of environmental stressors to become disordered whereas others can fall ill at minimal levels of stress.

THE PRIMACY OF EARLY EXPERIENCE: A CRITIQUE

The idea that early experiences shape personality and are strongly implicated in the development of clinical symptoms in adult life has been taken for granted by generations of psychotherapists. The theoretical assumption is that early learning must have a greater impact than later learning, because it occurs at a time when the organism is more plastic and when the child is more dependent on its parents. Many models also assume that the more severe the adult pathology, the earlier in childhood must be its origins.

In spite of their ubiquity, these ideas have not found support from empirical research. As discussed, developmental psychopathology shows that, by and large, negative events occurring early in life do *not*, by themselves, usually lead to psychiatric disorders. Given a reasonably favorable environment, most children will be resilient to stressful events. However, early stressors are often followed by later ones, so adversities that eventually become multiple and cumulative are more likely to begin early in development (Rutter 1989). How can we account for the cumulative effects of stressors? One possible explanation is that when too many things go wrong, children develop a sense that life events are outside their control. Another possible explanation is that continuous adversities overwhelm resilience mechanisms and prevent a child from recovering.

Why, then, do so many clinicians believe that earlier events are primary? Clearly, Sigmund Freud still has an influence. Moreover, therapists are, understandably, impressed by the narratives they hear from their patients. Moreover, many patients are influenced by their culture to believe that their problems must derive from dramatic childhood experiences. Clinical experience leads all too often to incorrect conclusions about cause and effect. The problem involves the invalidity of drawing broad conclusions from patient samples. What practitioners may fail to take into consideration is that many other individuals have had similar experiences to those of their patients and have become well-functioning adults in spite of them. Moreover, the negative effects of deprivations in *early* childhood can be counteracted by later, more positive experiences. For example, in a classical study of multifostered children, the effects of neglect and multiple separations were surprisingly reversible if the children were placed in a better environment in the school years (Clarke and Clarke 1979).

There is another important principle to keep in mind about the effects of early experience. Negative events in life are not independent but lead to each other in what have been called *developmental cascades* (Masten and Cicchetti 2010). For example, although most children are able to overcome family breakdown, losing a parent (usually a father) makes secondary consequences statistically more likely (McLanahan et al. 2013). The most important mediating factors in the outcome of family breakdown are financial distress or depression in the custodial parent and parental neglect, which then become risk factors in their own right. Without these developmental cascades, parental separation and loss in childhood would not consistently lead to adult psychopathology (Amato and Booth 1997).

To understand the impact of negative childhood experiences on the development of mental disorders, we must make a distinction between *risk factors* and *causal explanations*. In clinical epidemiology, risk factors are most likely to be etiological when they precede the development of pathology; when they are consistently, strongly, and specifically associated with the disorder; and when a plausible mechanism links the risk with the illness (Regier and Burke 1995). These criteria are rarely met in practice.

Associations between risk factors and disorders need not have any etiological significance. In some cases, an association can be statistically significant but account for only a small portion of the outcome of the variance. As Kraemer et al. (1997) noted: "It is difficult to find two variables that are absolutely independent of each other. Without considering some measure of potency in the assessment, given a large enough sample size, virtually every factor could be demonstrated to be a risk factor for every outcome that follows it" (p. 340). In other words, correlation does not prove causation. Associations between risks and disorders can often be accounted for other factors, termed *latent variables*. Many of these pathways involve gene-environment interactions. For example, negative experiences are more likely to occur to vulnerable children, particularly those whose difficult temperament makes it more difficult for their parents to achieve "goodness of fit" (Chess and Thomas 1984). Research has also shown that temperamentally difficult children are more likely to be maltreated by their parents (Rutter and Quinton 1984).

In summary, adverse life events in childhood increase the likelihood, above and beyond biological factors, of long-term psychopathological outcomes (Lippard and Nemeroff 2020). Yet, as I discuss later in this chapter, early life experiences of severe deprivation tend to have long-term effects in most, but not all cases. However, extreme circumstances are rare, and because so many nonpatients also have had adverse experiences, we cannot assume a simple cause-effect relationship between life events and psychopathology. The primacy of early experience is therefore a hypothesis that should be discarded—or at least regarded with great caution. It is inconsistent with a wide range of research in developmental psychology. This is not to say that early life experiences are not important or that they do not, in some cases, lead to long-term consequences, but it is another matter to assume they are the main cause of mental disorders or have a consistent relationship with them.

STRESS AND RESILIENCE

The prevalence of predispositions for psychopathology is certainly higher than the prevalence of any specific mental disorder. Fortunately, most people go through life carrying predispositions that are never expressed. In most cases, only severe and repeated stressors uncover these vulnerabilities. By definition, albeit a circular one, *stressful events* are those most likely to produce negative consequences. Stressors such as conflicts with parents during childhood or troubling life events can be idiosyncratic to the individual. Alternatively, they can consist of social or economic problems that affect everyone.

The literature is replete with evidence showing that adverse events during childhood have a relationship with adult psychopathology

(McLaughlin et al. 2010a, 2010b). On the other hand, negative events, particularly single events, need not produce long-term sequelae. Moreover, keep in mind that however strong the relationship between psychological risk factors and pathological outcome, it is statistical. Many are affected, but many are not. By and large, *resilience is the rule, not the exception*. This principle helps explain why only the most consistent adversities break down coping mechanisms. Multiple adversities lead to *stress sensitization* and are more likely to overcome resilience (Kendler et al. 2004).

One of the largest-scale studies of children at risk was a 30-year follow-up by Werner and Smith (1992). The sample was a cohort of children born to Hawaiian plantation workers. Although one might assume that poverty is a strong risk factor for developing mental disorders, this supposition was not confirmed by the findings. In fact, most of the children in the study eventually became fully competent adults. The effects of a stressful environment led to consistent sequelae only in a high-risk subgroup (10% of the total cohort). These children suffered from multiple adversities, such as dysfunction or breakup of the nuclear family or parental mental illness. In this subpopulation, the effect of environmental stressors was cumulative, showing a strong relationship between the *total number* of risk factors and the likelihood of a pathological outcome. About two-thirds of children with these multiple adversities eventually developed serious difficulties, most particularly learning problems, delinquency, or major mental disorders. Nevertheless, even in the high-risk group, as many as one-third became successful and competent. The most prominent traits that promoted resilience were an attractive personality, intelligence, persistence, a variety of interests, the capacity to be alone, and an optimistic approach to life. This study also demonstrated the interactions between the constitutional and environmental elements in resilience. Werner and Smith's cluster analysis of the protective influences on their cohort elicited four factors: 1) a temperamental nature that elicited caring responses; 2) an ability to develop realistic plans, regular working habits, and skills; 3) the presence of some degree of parental support; 4) availability of supportive adults outside the nuclear family. Although many of the children in this study had short-term difficulties during development, resilience was the rule in the long run. Thus, at adolescence, only one-third of those in the high-risk group were resilient, and two-thirds had problems, largely with conduct disorder. However, when the same cases were seen at age 30, most (five-sixths) of the troubled adolescents had become competent adults.

The conclusion that resilience is common in childhood has been confirmed in a large number of research studies all over the world (Goldstein and Brooks 2013). Resilience also emerges as a crucial factor determining the long-term effects of environmental stressors during adult life (Ong et al. 2009). As with other protective systems in the body, mental functioning can recover from adversity. Even the most severe stressors of adult life, such as war, terrorism, and natural disasters, only produce psychopathology in a minority of individuals (McNally 2003). As with children, effects of stress are cumulative in that the more negative events happen, the more likely the person is to develop symptoms. Research on the effects of life events, such as major transitions and changes, has shown that it is the cumulative weight of stressors that is related to medical illnesses and psychiatric disorders (Rahe 1995). Research on Vietnam veterans also confirms the clinical observation that the effects of trauma depend on severity of exposure (Dohrenwend et al. 2019). Finally, different people attach different valences to different events, depending on personality traits. This concept also corresponds to the principle of differential susceptibility to the environment (Belsky and Pluess 2009).

All these factors help explain why there are very few *specific* relationships between environmental stressors and psychiatric illness. The relationship between stress and most mental disorders is usually *nonspecific*. The same illness can be brought on by a variety of stressors, and the same stressors can bring on a wide variety of illnesses.

PERSONALITY, STRESS, AND RESILIENCE

Capacities intrinsic to the individual are the best predictors of successful coping throughout life. Personality traits are probably more useful than life events in predicting whether individuals develop mental disorders. In a well-known prospective research study on Harvard undergraduates followed throughout the life cycle (Vaillant 1977), the quality of childhood experience had little or no predictive value about the extent to which adults eventually achieved psychological maturity. Instead, school performance and defense styles (another way of assessing personality) were the best predictors of functioning in later life. In the same sample, McLaughlin et al. (2010a, 2010b) found that emotional reactivity—that is, a temperamental variation—was the best predictor of adult symptomatology. These findings point to the importance of interactions between childhood environment and adaptive functions. Although Harvard graduates are an unusual sample, DiRago and Vaillant (2007) replicated the findings in a longitudinal study of inner-city children that also followed its cohort over a lifetime. As the authors commented, "childhood environmental protector factors and parental social class predicted occupational status at age 25 significantly, but showed progressively weaker prediction at ages 32, 47, and 65. Timely early childhood development proved over time to be a far more important predictor than childhood social environment in adulthood" (p. 61).

Resilience to adversity may be ubiquitous when children find support outside the nuclear family, such as social supports in the extended family, in the schools, and in the community (Rutter 2012). However, the presence of favorable personality traits also makes it more likely that children at risk will be able to take advantage of these supports. Resilience is a mechanism that has passed through the sieve of natural selection. The mechanisms promoting psychological resilience make good sense in a Darwinian context; if people could not bounce back from adversity, life's inevitable traumas would interfere with fitness.

In summary, children are much tougher and more flexible than we usually think. This conclusion may be counterintuitive to readers who are accustomed to thinking that early childhood is a time of great vulnerability, but that is theory; the confirming evidence is not there. These conclusions do not imply that "everything is in the genes." Constitutional factors might be compared to a landscape through which a river of life events runs. Because life is often a chaotic process, the ultimate pattern resulting from this interaction is not predictable. However, the influence of life events will be influenced by the "lay of the land." Moreover, the environment of childhood is enormously complex. Risk factors interact with protective factors; therefore, only the most consistent adversities can deform personality functioning or produce symptoms.

Finally, there is no reason to believe that development and change ends in childhood or adolescence. Adult developmental theory, based on long-term prospective studies (e.g., Vaillant 2012) has shown that every stage of life presents its own demands and that people continue to change in respond to these challenges. Even a favorable childhood is no guarantee that people will remain happy later in development.

THE NATURE OF PSYCHOLOGICAL STRESSORS

Severe and repeated psychological stressors tend to be precursors or precipitants for the development of mental disorders. Longitudinal studies show that once a child is seriously off course, it is difficult to find the way back (see Chapter 4). In childhood, family dysfunction is the most common risk factor for adult psychopathology. This is probably because a dysfunctional family is a chronic stressor over many years and is often associated with more acutely stressful events. In adult life, the most common risks are the breakup of an intimate relationship and a serious problem at work. Each of these stressors can disrupt a life course and also lead to continuous sequelae over time.

As we have seen, behavioral genetic research shows that it is the unshared, and not the shared, environment that forms the crucial environmental contribution to most mental disorders. However, behavioral problems and emotional dysregulation are an exception, because they are also influenced by shared environmental factors deriving from families and neighborhoods (Rhee and Waldman 2002). However, some unshared variance may also derive from the family's reaction to a child's abnormal temperament (Pike et al. 1996).

TRAUMA, ABUSE, AND NEGLECT

Child abuse and neglect have been a central focus of environmental research in psychiatry and child development. These factors are clearly among the most powerful risks in childhood associated with adult psychopathology (Fergusson et al. 1996a, 1996b). Because it is dramatic and easier to document, child abuse (sexual or physical) has received the most attention, but abuse is often associated with physical or emotional neglect, sometimes combined with emotional abuse. These are generally continuous and could therefore be a stronger predictor of pathological outcomes.

The effects of neglect have also been studied in animal models. The best-known study was developed in research on rodents by my colleague at McGill, Michael Meaney. Rats who failed to provide sufficient maternal licking and grooming gave their offspring protection against environmental challenges, as shown by the offspring's level of stress hormones (glucocorticoids). Moreover, these effects also affect the epigenome and can be transmitted to future generations (Bagot et al. 2012: Meaney and Ferguson-Smith 2010).

Are these findings relevant to humans? Meaney's group has organized a prospective study of infants, the Maternal Adversity, Vulnerability, and Neurodevelopment (MAVAN) cohort to be followed over the course of their development. The study aims to show how children who are genetically sensitive to their environment react to different levels of care, much as was the case for rat pups. Thus far, results from this cohort have pointed to interactions between genes regulating serotonin and dopamine and the quality of early maternal care (Wazana et al. 2015). The effects of an adverse environment were also examined in a study of Holocaust survivor offspring. The finding was that parental PTSD had an effect on epigenetic coding in the next generation (Yehuda et al. 2014).

Human life is a bumpy road. Although resilience mechanisms function as a kind of psychological immune system, when stressors are persistent and severe, they can overwhelm these defenses. Some stressors do not appear problematic on the surface but exert subtle effects over time. One example is emotional neglect. This pattern can best be described as invalidating responses or failures to respond to emotional distress in a child. Linehan (1993) posited invalidation as the main environmental factor leading to borderline personality disorder (BPD). Emotional neglect can have a lasting effect on those whose emotions are intense and unstable.

A good deal of research has focused on child abuse, which can be physical or sexual. Parental responses to children can also be directly hurtful, in which case we can speak of emotional abuse. A relationship definitely exists between all these risk factors and psychopathology in children (Jaffee 2017). However, the idea that physically abused children grow up to be violent and tend to abuse their own children turns out, as shown by longitudinal research, not to be true (Widom 1989). Longitudinal follow-up of a cohort whose maltreatment (abuse or neglect) was severe enough to come to the attention of the courts showed that about one-third developed PTSD (Widom 1999), whereas about 15% developed BPD (Widom et al. 2009).

Our own research group (Laporte et al. 2011) found that sisters, one of whom had BPD, were rarely concordant for this disorder, in spite of growing up in the same family and reporting the same experiences. It follows that although child abuse and neglect are risk factors for adult psychopathology, one cannot assume that abused and neglected children will develop a particular mental disorder. It also does not follow that patients with disorders in which childhood trauma is frequent will necessarily have abuse histories.

A useful test of the idea that severity and chronicity of adversity can overwhelm defenses comes from research on Romanian orphans. The largest study was conducted in the United Kingdom under the leadership of Michael Rutter, who described this data as a "natural experiment" (Rutter et al. 2012). The cohort was a group of newborns placed in poorly managed orphanages, where basic needs received little attention. The findings of longitudinal follow-up to adulthood in this cohort have been published (Sonuga-Barke et al. 2017) and showed that the sooner children were adopted (before 6 months), with a shorter time in the orphanage, the better they did later. Although differences between groups with shorter or longer stays were not large at age 11, they increased in young adulthood (ages 22–25 years), with effects on symptoms of autism spectrum disorder, disinhibited social engagement, inattention and overactivity, cognitive impairment, low educational achievement, unemployment, and use of mental health services. Although most of those who had been in the orphanages for more than 6 months showed some degree of impairment, however, about 20% were not impaired. Thus, even in this natural experiment, resilience played some role.

It was also reported that the presence of the long allele of the serotonin transporter gene (*5HTT*) reduced the risk of long-term consequences (Kumsta et al. 2010). Although a single polymorphism is unlikely to account for a large percentage of the variance, a gene that reduces the level of reaction of stress could be protective. This is not to deny that severe adversities, particularly if they begin early in life and continues for some time, can negatively affect children later on. Stressors in adult life also can produce permanent damage. One example is the Holocaust (Sharon et al. 2009), as documented in a large community study in Israel in which more than 15% had anxiety disorders and more than 60% experienced insomnia. However, the subjects did not have higher rates of depression and PTSD. Thus, even under conditions of maximum adversity, most adults do not develop severe psychopathology later in life.

SOCIAL STRESSORS

The most important stressors in childhood do not all arise from experiences in the family (Harris 2009). A good deal of evidence suggests that peer groups, neighborhood factors, and socioeconomic status also contribute to psychopathology. These findings are not always taken into consideration by clinicians.

Stressors derived from the wider social sphere can affect virtually everyone. For example, poverty is associated with psychopathology, and as shown by Wilkinson and Pickett (2009), overall health in the population is predicted by high levels of economic inequality. In the well-known Whitehall study (Marmot et al. 1991), workers in the British government attained better health if they were high in the work hierarchy and had worse health if they were low in that hierarchy. Unemployment is generally more stressful than problems on the job. Long-term trends over many decades have shown that more people are admitted to mental hospitals when unemployment is high than when it is low (Brenner 1973).

Many mental disorders have strikingly different levels of prevalence in different socioeconomic levels and different cultural settings (Kirmayer 2006; Murphy 1982). The prevalence of mental disorders can also change rapidly over time, producing cohort effects that reflect changes in social structures and demands (Robins and Regier 1991). For example, the prevalence of antisocial behavior and suicide went up after the Second World War and then declined (Rutter and Smith 1995). By lowering the threshold of liability, social factors can change the prevalence of these disorders dramatically within a single generation. Social factors can determine whether people who lose a job are able to find another one. Even the availability of intimacy could depend on these factors, because individuals with a strong social network have a better chance of finding (or replacing) a partner.

CONCLUSION

In summary, only the most complex relationships between multiple genetic and multiple environmental factors account for the pathways to mental illness. The relationship between risks and disorders in psychiatry is therefore *nonlinear*. We can be exposed to many risk factors without falling ill. This is because personality traits, like an immune system, make us vulnerable to psychopathology or protect us against mental illness. However, at some point natural defenses can be overwhelmed. Mental disorders then become relatively independent of the risk factors that produced them. This is why psychopathology sometimes emerges like ketchup from a bottle—either not at all, or all at once.

CHAPTER 4

GENE-ENVIRONMENT INTERACTIONS

THE GENE-ENVIRONMENT MODEL

Gene-environment interactions are the key to understanding the complex origins of most mental disorders.

Psychiatrists of my generation always knew that schizophrenia and bipolar disorder cannot develop without biological vulnerability. What we had not been taught is that virtually *all* forms of psychopathology are associated with heritable predispositions. We were also not taught that even when biological factors are strong, psychosocial risks still have a role to play. Thus, the impact of life events cannot be understood without taking genetics and temperament into account, and the impact of constitutional vulnerability cannot be understood without considering the effect of life stressors. You cannot account for psychopathology unless you consider how genes interact with environments.

A predisposition-stress (or stress-diathesis) model in psychiatry has a long history (Monroe and Simons 1991). The most influential advocate of this idea in the previous century was the Swiss-American psychiatrist Adolf Meyer (Muncie 1939). George Engel's (1980) "biopsychosocial model" of mental disorders revived and modernized the principles of Meyerian psychiatry, hypothesizing that mental disorders emerge from interactions between biological, psychological, and social risk (and protective) factors. The biopsychosocial model encouraged psychiatrists to think multidimensionally. However, such a model may still be too simple, given the vast interactions between multiple risk factors. A more recent way of formulating mental disorders, while avoiding either biological or psychosocial reductionism, has been called a *network model*, an approach that has had increasing influence in biology and psychology generally (Borsboom et al. 2019).

In light of these complexities, it is worth keeping mind that there is no direct path from risk to disorder in individual patients. Moreover, the same diatheses that can lead to illness can also lead to better-than-average mental health (Belsky and Pluess 2009). Thus, when we make "formulations" about patients, we are not making predictions, but post-dictions.

Consider the difference between the necessary and sufficient conditions for developing psychopathology. *Necessary conditions* are those without which a mental disorder cannot develop. Heritable predispositions tend to be necessary causes for mental disorders but only become sufficient when people are also exposed to environmental stressors. (This is what medicine calls a "double-hit model.") Usually, multiple stressors will be involved, each of which contributes to a cumulative effect that crosses a threshold of liability. *Sufficient conditions* would be those in whose presence a disorder inevitably develops. In principle, these could consist of the interactive and cumulative effects of genes and environment. Because most diseases have multiple causes, only a complex combination of necessary risk factors can ever be "sufficient." That is why we cannot accurately predict the development of mental disorders.

Risk factors do not produce pathology on their own but have different effects in vulnerable individuals, in whom a small amount of stress can precipitate a severe illness. Moreover, similar clinical outcomes can emerge from different etiological pathways, or what Cicchetti (1995) called "equifinality." Thus, some patients with a disorder have stronger predispositions, leading them to become ill at low levels of exposure to stress. Other patients with the same disorder have weaker predispositions, becoming ill only when exposed to high levels of stress. Moreover, the same risks can lead to different outcomes, or what Cicchetti called "multifinality" (Cicchetti and Rogosch 1996). Thus, the same life events can lead to entirely different outcomes in different individuals. Finally, illnesses often show differences in course or symptomatology that tend to depend on the strength of genetic predispositions. Genes also determine the thresholds for developing specific psychiatric disorders and shape wider spectrum of outcomes, ranging from overt illness to differences in personality. One well-known example is the relationship of schizotypal personality traits to the psychotic symptoms of schizophrenia (Meehl 1990).

The relationship between traits and disorders is a crucial aspect of the model. Individuals may have genetically determined traits without ever developing any of the disorders associated with them. Thus, for every person who falls ill, many others who have the same traits will never develop a disorder. In many forms of mental illness, the environment is the primary determinant of whether people cross the threshold of liability between trait and disorder.

Let us consider, as an illustration, an example from medicine in which mechanisms are well known: the etiology of tuberculosis. Although infectious diseases cannot develop without the presence of a specific organism, most individuals who have the bacterium causing tuberculosis in their lungs never develop an illness. Therefore, the infectious agent is a necessary but not a sufficient cause of disease. Many other factors, most particularly genetic predispositions to infection affecting the immune system, as well as environmental factors such as nutrition and poverty, determine whether illness will develop (Childs et al. 1992). Tuberculosis becomes clinically apparent only when the cumulative effects of all these risks cross a threshold.

Similar mechanisms apply to mental disorders.

Genes and environment can interact via several mechanisms (Kendler and Eaves 1986; Rutter 2006). The first involves *additive* genetic and environmental effects. That is our usual way of thinking about the subject—genes raise the liability to a certain degree, after which environmental risks further increase it, and psychopathology develops when the total liability crosses a threshold. However, some gene-environment effects are nonlinear; a small increase in risk can produce a large effect on outcome.

A second mechanism involves genetic control of *susceptibility* to the environment. In other words, individuals differ in the extent to which they experience life events as stressful. This has been described by the concept of *differential sensitivity* (Belsky and Pluess 2009).

A third mechanism involves genetic control of *exposure* to the environment. In this case, individuals with given traits will be more likely to act in a way that exposes them to adverse environmental influences. For example, a difficult child is more likely to suffer from rejection.

These mechanisms can also be described as *gene-environment correlations*, which can be further subdivided (Rutter 2006). *Passive correlations* occur when parents who pass on problematic genes also create problematic environments for children. *Active correlations* occur when the traits of a child lead to selection of a particular kind of environment. *Evocative correlations* occur when the behavior of a child shapes responses from family, peers, or other people in their environment.

Personality traits influence both exposure to and susceptibility to environmental stressors. This is why some individuals are much more likely than others to be exposed to negative life events. One example is that adults with an impulsive temperament are much more likely to get into trouble with other people, resulting in job loss or interpersonal rejection. Genetic control of exposure to the environment means that predispositions influence both the severity and the frequency of negative life events.

Individual differences in susceptibility mean that personality traits can make individuals more vulnerable to negative life events. For example, those who score high on the personality dimension of neuroticism are more likely to put a pessimistic "spin" on various life events. Those who are more dependent on social approval and the support of significant others are more likely to be devastated by rejections or losses, whereas those who are temperamentally less responsive to the reactions of others will be less affected.

People can experience the same events as negative, positive, or neutral; thus, we cannot assess the effects of life events without considering how they are processed. The fact that the same environmental stressors produce different effects on different people is also one of the reasons for the lack of concordance in personality or psychological symptoms between siblings. Years ago, Plomin (1990) pointed out that measures of the environment used by psychologists in which people filled out questionnaires tell us as much about heritable traits as about what actually happened in their lives.

Siblings growing up in the same family who are treated much in the same way end up being almost as different from each other as perfect strangers (Dunn and Plomin 1990). This observation is well known to parents. It has been said that mothers with one child believe in the environment, whereas mothers with two children come to believe in the genes.

That life events have a genetic component may be surprising to those who assume that the environment is an external force. Yet the list of events that are heritable is rather long and includes marital problems, divorce, friendships, social supports, problems at work, socioeconomic status, and education, all of which have heritability ranging between 30% and 50% (Plomin 2018).

In summary, life events are *not* random or external to the individual. Although there *is* such a thing as good or bad luck in life, personality determines how likely we are to be exposed to negative events, as well as our ultimate response to them. Some suffer more than their share of life's vicissitudes. Others seem to have "a charmed life," either because they avoid being exposed to stress or because they emerge from adversity relatively unscathed.

One of the most important ideas to emerge in recent research has been the difference between people who are profoundly affected by even small changes in the environment and those for whom adversity can be more or less shrugged off. Boyce (2019) has referred to these trait patterns as "orchids" and "dandelions." This is the same concept as differential sensitivity to the environment (Belsky and Pluess 2009). Boyce's research has shown that most people are dandelions, in that it takes a severe stressor to create serious consequences for them. In contrast, a minority (about 15%) are orchids, who tend to fall victim to mental disorders (but can also have unusually productive lives) (Boyce 2019).

Examples of gene-environment interaction have been documented in the research literature. One is the effects of child maltreatment, which are more likely to lead to psychopathology, particularly conduct disorder, in those who are genetically sensitive to trauma (Jaffee 2017; Tabery 2014; Uher and Zwicker 2017). Some of the same mechanisms affect the response to adult trauma, as in the genetic predispositions that make PTSD more likely in adults (True et al. 1993).

LONGITUDINAL STUDIES OF BIRTH COHORTS

I now review some of the research designs that might provide empirical support for gene-environment models of mental disorder.

Longitudinal research following children into adulthood opens the possibility of being able to observe the early signs of mental disorder. However, few studies have included genetic measures that allow for the assessment of gene-environment interactions.

Cohen et al. (2005) conducted the Children in the Community (CIC) Study, following about 800 children growing up in the Albany-Saratoga region of New York State through their adult years. The study was able to demonstrate that mental disorders associated with suicidality, violence, or problematic relationships have identifiable markers early in development and that many of these are related to personality traits that put people at risk for personality disorders. (However, not enough subjects developed symptoms meeting standard criteria for the diagnosis of specific personality disorders.) Another large-scale project following children into adulthood was the Great Smoky Mountains Study (Costello et al. 2016).

While these were landmark studies, their findings could not demonstrate causality. Moreover, it is better to start longitudinal research at infancy rather than at school age. One way to address this obstacle is to use birth cohorts, following groups of children born at the same time so that measurements can be made early in development.

Several of these studies were conducted in the United Kingdom: the National Survey of Health and Development, started in 1946 (Wadsworth et al. 2006); the National Child Development Study, started in 1958 (Power and Elliott 2006); the 1970 British Cohort Study (Elliott and Shepherd 2006); and the Millennium Cohort Study from 2000 (Connelly and Platt 2014). Each of these cohorts included between 15,000 and 20,000 children. Another study with a similar sample was the Avon Longitudinal Study of Parents and Children (Golding and ALSPAC Study Team 2004). On the continent, the World Health Organization sponsored the European Longitudinal Study of Pregnancy and Childhood (Golding 1989).

All these birth cohort studies have provided large amounts of data on the frequency of depression as well as antisocial behavior, depression, and the risk factors for these outcomes. However, this kind of data cannot distinguish between the genetic and environmental precursors of mental disorders. That requires a different research design.

THE DUNEDIN STUDY

If researchers can measure biological and/or genetic markers in adults, then birth cohort studies could use that data to measure gene-environment interactions. The problem is that this method is limited by our rather primitive ability to measure these markers. Nonetheless, one study of this kind has had major impact.

The Dunedin Multidisciplinary Health and Development Study is a birth cohort of more than 1,000 children born between 1972 and 1973 in New Zealand (Poulton et al. 2015). There was an advantage in collecting a sample from a small city where people are less likely to move around. (This is why Michael Rutter conducted his largest study in the Isle of Wight and why the Czech-born psychiatrist Rudolph Uher works in Nova Scotia.) Moreover, researchers have been able to track these subjects even when they did move far away. The results of the Dunedin study have had a major impact on developmental psychopathology. They were also the subject of a television series a few years ago (*Why Am I?: The Science of Us* [New Zealand, 2016]).

The most widely cited reports from the Dunedin cohort emerged under the leadership of the husband and wife team of Avshalom Caspi and Terrie Moffitt, who are now at Duke University. Caspi and Moffitt spent several years in London and have often collaborated with Rutter, with whom they authored a useful review of the entire field (Rutter et al. 2006).

Two papers published by this team (Caspi et al. 2002, 2003) have been among the most quoted in all of psychology, with thousands of citations (the 2003 paper on depression has almost 9,000). Their findings are considered foundational in the study of gene-environment interactions in psychopathology. Their 2002 paper on antisocial behavior and the 2003 paper on depression reported that although genetic risks and environmental risks, by themselves, do not necessarily raise the risk for mental disorders, the combination of both does so significantly. In each case, they selected a genetic locus already known to be associated to some extent with a specific outcome. Caspi et al. (2002) examined a polymorphism of the monoamine oxidase gene (*MAO*), which, when combined with maltreatment, predicted antisocial behavior. Caspi et al. (2003) found that when stressful life events occurred in individuals with one or two copies of the short allele of the serotonin *5-HTT* promoter polymorphism, they developed more depression than individuals homozygous for the long allele.

Although these observations are now 20 years old, they continue to stir up controversy. The findings on antisocial behavior have been replicated using three genetic loci instead of one (Cicchetti et al. 2012). A 30-year longitudinal study of 398 males (in a birth cohort from Christchurch, New Zealand) supported the model (Fergusson et al. 2011a, 2011b). The relationship was also supported by a meta-analysis of 27 studies (Byrd and Manuck 2014). Yet for other researchers, the findings seem difficult to replicate, especially those pertaining to the relationship to depression (e.g., Peyrot et al. 2018). A meta-analysis did not support the Caspi group's (2002) findings (Culverhouse et al. 2018). Another failure of replication for depression comes from the same longitudinal study that supported findings for antisocial behavior (Fergusson et al. 2011a), which failed to support the link between depression, childhood trauma, and the gene *5-HTTLPR* that controls serotonergic activity. Moreover, *5-HTTLPR* has no relationship to depression in genome-wide association studies (Border et al. 2019).

One reason why this debate is still open after 20 years of research is most probably the complexity of the variables under study. First, it is unlikely a single gene, even in interaction with life adversities, can explain a large percentage of variance. Results can be statistically significant in a large sample but may not account for a large percentage of the outcome. Second, the psychological variables under study are complex: as is discussed in Chapter 8, major depression is a heterogeneous construct.

This story underlies an important complication: genetic and environmental risk factors do not follow the categorical system of diagnosis in the DSM manuals, but are *transdiagnostic*. Researchers have identified a common element in all forms of psychopathology, called the *psychopathology factor*, or *p factor* (Caspi and Moffitt 2018; Caspi et al. 2014).

LONGITUDINAL STUDIES OF TWINS

Following twins (both monozygotic and dizygotic) longitudinally over time allows researchers to control for genetic effects and to measure interactions with the environment. This is an expensive but probably indispensable way to separate the effects of genes and environment.

One of the best known of these cohorts is the Minnesota Twin Family Study, begun in 1983, consisting of 8,000 twin pairs who entered the study between ages 11 and 17 years (Krueger and Johnson 2002). One part of the study made headlines by finding that monozygotic twins separated at birth were surprisingly similar in behavior. The cohort has been used to follow adolescents with borderline personality disorder, estimating the effects of genes and environment at different stages of development (Bornovalova et al. 2013).

Twin cohort studies have also been initiated in other countries, including a Chinese cohort of 2,000 pairs (Tong et al. 2018) and several cohorts in Scandinavia. However, the richest source of data relevant to psychiatry from samples in the community has been the Virginia Twin Study of Adolescent Behavioral Development, led by Kenneth Kendler at Virginia Commonwealth University, using data from 2,762 families (Kendler and Prescott 2006). A similar project in the United Kingdom, the Environmental Risk Longitudinal Twin Study, has been following a sample of twins born in 1994–95 (Hannon et al. 2018). Many of the details of findings from these studies will be referenced in chapters related to specific disorders. By and large, they confirm what we already know from behavioral genetics—that mental disorders have a strong heritable component—but we are just at the beginning of this research program.

EPIGENETICS

Epigenetics is a hot topic in biological research. The principle is that life experiences, while not changing the genome itself, produce changes in genetic switches (methyl groups or histones) that turn genes on and off or act as a dimmer switch. Moreover, these changes can be passed on to future generations. This effect was shown in a study of the 1944–45 Dutch famine, in which epigenetic markers can be found in the grandchildren of those who were exposed to severe hunger (Heijmans et al. 2008). Epigenetics also helps explain why monozygotic twins are not fully "identical," either in utero or as they grow older.

The most widely quoted study of epigenetics was conducted in rats by a team led by my McGill colleague Michael Meaney (Weaver et al. 2004). This report showed that effects of higher rates of licking and grooming of pups in the early weeks of life persisted into adulthood. Although this model could be interpreted as supporting the psychodynamic idea that personality and behavior can be shaped by early experience, that is a stretch. The same research group found that people who had died by suicide and had earlier reported childhood abuse had less expression of hippocampal glucocorticoid receptors than did nonabused subjects who died from suicide or nonsuicidal subjects. However, this study, unlike the one in rats, was not longitudinal but depended on the validity of childhood memories.

These studies have aroused great interest, particularly in the neuroscience community, but the breadth of applicability of epigenetic mechanisms remains unknown. I once heard a neuroscientist at a conference thank Dr. Meaney for "bringing us to pay attention to the environment." However, we should have been paying attention all along.

THE THRESHOLD MODEL OF DISEASE

Most of us usually consider people as either sick or well and are accustomed to thinking of health and illness as a dichotomy. Yet in most cases, a *continuum* between health and illness eixsts. We all carry around with us a set of liabilities, genetic potentials to develop specific diseases, that become activated in the presence of stressful environmental factors. Thus, predispositions caused by multiple genes are quantitative and lead to a *continuous* distribution of variations, with no sharp break between predisposing traits and disorders. This complexity creates continuity between health and illness, depending on how many pathogenic genes are activated, the weight of biological predispositions, and the strength of environmental stressors. These weights vary from one person to another: some individuals with a stronger genetic weighting can develop illness with little or no environmental provocation, whereas others with weaker predispositions may only develop illness if exposed to severe adversity.

A familiar clinical example of this principle is hypertension. Multiple genes are involved in the predisposition to this disease (Falconer and Mackay 1996). Moreover, many environmental factors, ranging from diet to kidney disease, can raise blood pressure. These environmental effects will be much more pathogenic in those who are genetically pre-disposed to hypertension. The traditional cutoff for hypertension (blood pressure 140/90) simply reflects our clinical experience that, some-where around this point, the secondary complications of hypertension become much more likely. As is shown later chapters, a number of psy-chiatric conditions are based on traits that have crossed a threshold at which they are more likely to produce significant dysfunction.

The threshold model of disease can be modeled mathematically to sum all qualitative factors, genetic and environmental, that contribute to the expression of a trait, creating a continuously distributed quanti-tative measure termed *liability*. Certain observable characteristics of dis-ease help determine the nature of liability. The first concerns the natural history of an illness. Some genetic predispositions have "sleeper" ef-fects that only become manifest later in life. (The genetic predisposition to Alzheimer's disease is one example.) Another is the relationship be-tween age at onset and the strength of genetic weighting. Early onset cases tend to have a larger genetic component, whereas late-onset cases tend to have a larger environmental component. Early onset cases tend to have more affected relatives and be more severe, whereas late-onset cases tend to have fewer affected relatives and be less severe. Childs and Scriver (1986) offered illustrations of the principle that age at onset is a marker for the strength of a genetic predisposition. In a variety of chronic diseases, an early age at onset is associated with a stronger family his-tory and more severe illness.

A second feature that could be used as a marker for predispositions is sex distribution. Childs and Scriver (1982) suggested that when an ill-ness has a skewed sex distribution, then the sex affected less frequently by a disease will have a stronger family history and be more severe. This is because when genetic factors are relatively sex limited, they de-velop in interaction with hormones. In the absence of hormonal factors, they must have greater penetrance. For example, although systemic lu-pus erythematosus is more common in females, it is more severe and has a stronger family history in males. In the same way, gout is more common in males but is more severe and has a stronger family history in females. Mental disorders with a skewed sex distribution, such as de-pression and substance abuse in adults as well as several common psy-chiatric disorders of childhood, show a parallel relationship between sex and strength of liability.

Multiple thresholds for the same disease can occur when the illness has more severe and less severe subtypes (McGuffin and Gottesman 1985). Multiple thresholds can also be interpreted as indicating two path-ways to the same illness, each involving a different weight of genetic loading. The best example in psychiatry is depression, in which the melancholic and psychotic subtypes have different patterns of predispositions and stressors from less severe forms.

Thus, the threshold for any disease is not fixed but is sensitive to the environment. Even in single-gene diseases, like phenylketonuria, the predisposition causes severe disease with one type of diet but no disease at all with another type of diet. This principle applies with even greater force to multiple-gene diseases. The same environmental stressors that lead to chronic illness in one person will lead to acute illness in a second person and to no illness in a third person.

The large difference between the twin and molecular estimates (a "heritability gap" or "missing heritability") shows that we cannot, at this point, translate the data from behavior genetics into molecular terms. This is why the optimism of 20 years ago needs to be replaced with humility and patience. However, what researchers may have forgotten is that genetic factors in mental disorders have little meaning or predictive value outside of the context of development and psychosocial factors.

REDUCTIONISM AND EMERGENCE IN GENE-ENVIRONMENT INTERACTION

Over the past several centuries, science has benefited from strategies to break down complex phenomena into more manageable components. In philosophy, this is called *reductionism* (Godfrey-Smith 2014). Reductionism has been a success in science up to now, but it may not be sufficient to understand the most complex systems in nature.

We can work our way down a hierarchy of concepts to a level that is believed to be fundamental. In neuroscience, this often means understanding behavior in terms of the activity and connections and neurons. This idea is reflected in the development of the Research Domain Criteria (Cuthbert and Insel 2013), which aim to account for psychopathology as abnormal neuroconnectivity. However, something crucial is lost when we fail to study the world at "higher" levels of analysis. The whole may be greater than the sum of its parts. Characteristics at the level of a person or an organism may not be fully explained by reduction to a cellular level. For example, water has features that are not explained by its components (hydrogen and oxygen). This is even more true of highly complex systems. The concept that complexity produces new, nonreducible phenomena is called *emergence* (Corning 2002).

As we have seen, genetic effects on behavioral traits and psychopathology are extremely complex. Combine that with a vast range of interacting environmental factors, and you have a system of incredible complexity. It is extraordinarily naïve to think that we can understand human behavior in terms of the genome or the neuron. Unfortunately, our minds crave simplicity, and researchers have been seduced by the wish to explain mental disorders by derangements in chemistry and neurotransmission.

CONCLUSION

Uher and Zwicker (2017) had a nicely balanced view of these challenges:

> Intriguing findings on genetic and environmental causation suggest a need to reframe the etiology of mental disorders. Molecular genetics shows that thousands of common and rare genetic variants contribute to mental illness. Epidemiological studies have identified dozens of environmental exposures that are associated with psychopathology. The effect of environment is likely conditional on genetic factors, resulting in gene-environment interactions. The impact of environmental factors also depends on previous exposures, resulting in environment-environment interactions. Most known genetic and environmental factors are shared across multiple mental disorders. Schizophrenia, bipolar disorder and major depressive disorder, in particular, are closely causally linked. Synthesis of findings from twin studies, molecular genetics and epidemiological research suggests that joint consideration of multiple genetic and environmental factors has much greater explanatory power than separate studies of genetic or environmental causation. Multi-factorial gene-environment interactions are likely to be a generic mechanism involved in the majority of cases of mental illness, which is only partially tapped by existing gene-environment studies. (p. 121)

Clearly, the study of gene-environment interactions is just beginning. We need more research to examine both sources of variance in the same populations.

CHAPTER 5

▬ DIAGNOSES, DISORDERS, AND TRAITS

TO SORT out the role of nature and nurture in mental disorders, we need to know whether the current system for diagnosing these disorders is valid. This chapter discusses problems and limitations in the criteria used in the DSM classification of mental disorders as well as the relationship between underlying traits and diagnosable disorders.

LIMITS OF THE DSM SYSTEM

I am old enough to have used every edition of DSM, from the first to the fifth. Although each revision has highlighted important clinical issues, psychiatry is held back by its inability (with a few exceptions) to understand what causes mental illness. The DSM classification is almost entirely based on symptoms, and as long as that is the case, it can never be fully valid. The situation in most other areas of medicine is different; most diseases are defined on the basis of etiology and pathogenesis. That is why the categorization of medical illnesses changes more slowly. Physicians who attended medical school 50 years ago will find that the names of most diseases remain the same. In contrast, the classification of psychiatric disorders has changed dramatically over time. Again, the problem is that mental disorders are defined on the basis of phenomenology. In other words, DSM categories are syndromes, not diseases.

In principle, it was a wise decision to replace the DSM-I (American Psychiatric Association 1952) and DSM-II (American Psychiatric Association 1968) classifications, based on dubious causal models, with the relatively atheoretical schema introduced in DSM-III (American Psychiatric

Association 1980). However, the categories in that edition and the current version, DSM-5 (American Psychiatric Association 2013), can only be provisional. They provide a common language for clinicians but are not based on a deeper knowledge of etiology and pathogenesis. The problem is that once a diagnosis appears in the manual, it is treated as though it were as valid as congestive heart failure. When DSM-III came out, it presented its system as being, at least potentially, reliable and valid. Although its limitations were obvious, it was expected that further research would sharpen diagnosis to the point of being able to find links to etiological factors and make predictions of treatment response. That is not what happened.

In many ways, we are no further ahead today than we were in 1980 (Paris 2015a). Although DSM-5 had been initially proposed as a paradigm shift that would introduce a dimensional system of diagnosis, the evidence was not sufficient to justify such a radical change. Thus, although the task force that oversaw the writing of the manual had originally wanted disorders reclassified using quantitative dimensional scores, this system was only applied to personality disorders, and even that schema remains in Section III of DSM-5 (diagnoses that require further study).

However, there are proposals in the literature to replace categories with dimensional scores. The Hierarchical Taxonomy of Psychopathology (HiTOP) aims to dimensionalize *all* psychiatric diagnoses (Kotov et al. 2015), but this system is also not likely to be adopted without major support from research. As one of my colleagues reminded the authors of HiTOP at a recent convention, we have had dimensional measures of psychopathology (such as the Minnesota Multiphasic Personality Inventory) for many decades, but none has replaced categorical diagnosis.

It is true that categories can be arbitrary compared with quantitative spectra. However, the human mind is designed to think about phenomena using a yes/no framework. That is one reason why medicine as a whole continues to prefer categories for diagnosis. Psychiatry would be taking an enormous risk to replace all its categories with dimensions, effectively blowing up the bridge to the rest of medicine that it laboriously rebuilt some 50 years ago. If we knew the etiology of major mental disorders, we could return to categories and be comfortable with them, but many psychiatrists feel disappointed by the lack of progress in research to make classification more valid. (As we have seen, we were promised a breakthrough once the human genome was sequenced, but that did not happen.) In the long run, psychiatry remains committed to converting its current symptom-based system into a schema rooted in biological mechanisms, but this is a task for another century of research.

The complexity of the human brain is the main obstacle in our way, but it is also possible that modern neuroscience is not up to the challenge because it is based on the wrong assumptions. This is where the nature-nurture problem comes again in view. Psychiatrists who believe that behavior, feelings, and thoughts are "nothing but" vagaries in the functioning of neurons are adopting what has been called a *biomedical model* and tend to practice like internists. Their patients are treated almost entirely with drugs, often leading to problematic polypharmacy. Thus, taking the nature side of nature versus nurture creates a reductionistic theory associated with a simplistic approach to practice that all too often fails. This approach to psychiatry is, however, consistent in many ways with the DSM system, which is based on symptoms and has been interpreted in a way that sees them as targets for pharmacological intervention.

Similarly, psychiatrists who believe that psychopathology is "nothing but" a reexperiencing and reenactment of past life adversities, or a reflection of problematic cognitive schemas, will also practice in a simplistic mode. In this case, taking the nurture side of the debate may mean that DSM diagnoses are taken much less seriously than they deserve.

Another problem with the DSM system is that the boundaries around its categories are fuzzy. In fact, most of the diagnoses in DSM describe heterogeneous populations of patients. Imprecision is built into a system that allows diagnoses to meet just more than half of the written criteria. As a result, categories overlap with each other, and most patients require multiple diagnoses to account for their symptoms. The high levels of comorbidity in clinical populations are nothing but an artifact of the diagnostic system (Jensen and Hoagwood 1997).

The comorbidity promoted by the DSM system is a serious problem for psychiatric research. Multiple diagnoses are particularly common in the patients we most need to study—those with the most severe levels of dysfunction (Kessler et al. 1994). We have to cope with a system that promotes fuzzy categories and is unable to provide superordinate diagnoses that could account for multiple sectors of dysfunction.

At best, even if DSM fails to reflect a coherent etiological model for understanding psychopathology, it provides us with a common language for clinical practice and research. This is why, in spite of all these problems, I have used the DSM classification to guide the organization of the chapters in this book.

DETERMINING DIAGNOSTIC VALIDITY

Fifty years ago, a group of psychiatrists at Washington University in St. Louis, supported by Robert Spitzer at Columbia University in New York, convinced psychiatry that it needed a classification that was both reliable and valid. Led by Eli Robins and Samuel Guze, they described five basic criteria for the validity of any psychiatric diagnosis: 1) precise clinical description; 2) laboratory studies identifying biological markers; 3) clear delimitation from other disorders; 4) a characteristic outcome in follow-up studies; and 5) a genetic pattern in family history studies (Robins and Guze 1970). None of the major psychiatric disorders meet all of these criteria. Many of the present categories remain *clinically* useful, in that they describe entities that most practitioners recognize and can agree on, thus providing tools for communication between clinicians. We are used to DSM diagnoses but should not believe they are "real."

A series of field trials conducted along with the development of DSM-5 was rather discouraging. Even major depression, often seen as the best-researched diagnosis in the manual, failed to attain adequate reliability, and the kappa between observers was only 0.2 (Regier et al. 2013). However, as shown later in this book, this finding was hardly surprising given the lack of demarcation between depression as a disorder and unhappiness as a state of mind.

TRAITS, DISORDERS, AND ADAPTATION

If there is continuous variation between normality and pathology, it should also not be surprising that we have difficulty classifying mental disorders into discrete entities. If categories are not real entities, we should expect to find sharp boundaries between them. Instead, many mental disorders can be better understood as extreme points on a continuum.

What is inherited when there is a genetic vulnerability to psychopathology? When we think in terms of natural selection, it seems to make no sense for *any* mental illness to be inherited! The only way to understand this paradox is to assume that what is genetically transmitted is not a disorder but a *trait*. These are characteristics that can be adaptive under one set of circumstances and maladaptive under another set. This helps to explain why, even in the presence of predispositions, heritability need not be expressed unless environmental stressors are present. This model is perfectly compatible with Darwinian natural selection, as well as with the hypothesis that mental disorders reflect aberrations in hardwired evolutionary programs. Several books have outlined a Darwinian approach to the etiology of mental disorders (Brune 2015; McGuire and Troisi 1998; Nesse 2019; Nesse and Williams 1995; Stevens and Price 2000). The idea behind these models is that most mental disorders are maladaptive variants of adaptive mechanisms. This principle cannot, however, be applied universally. In some cases, mental disorders demonstrate sharp qualitative breaks from normality (as is the case for schizophrenia.)

There are also problems associated with seeing diagnosis as continuous with normality. *Diagnostic inflation* (Frances 2013; Paris 2015a) results from failing to draw these boundaries. The most common examples in recent years have been overdiagnosis of major depression, bipolar disorder, generalized anxiety disorder, ADHD, and autism spectrum disorders. Each has a fuzzy boundary with normal phenomena, such as sadness, moodiness, inattentiveness, social ineptness, and worry. The DSM system has encouraged physicians to identify all these conditions as mental disorders, leading to many false positives (Paris 2015b). The result is that the concept of normality is being lost and diagnoses long considered rare have become common (Frances 2013). This muddying of the diagnostic waters could have an unfortunate effect on research into the conditions that everyone recognizes to be abnormal and pathological. As I discuss in Chapter 8, the conflation of normal sadness with melancholic depression has seriously set back our understanding of severe cases of mood disorder.

RESEARCH DOMAIN CRITERIA SYSTEM

The National Institute of Mental Health (NIMH) has developed the Research Domain Criteria (RDoC) as a guide to future research, with the hope that it could eventually lead to a substitute for current diagnostic methods in psychiatry by filling the gap between categories and biological endophenotypes (Cuthbert and Insel 2013). RDoC aims to be based on neuroscience, focusing on abnormal neural connectivity. As of 2013, to apply for research grants at NIMH, investigators have been advised to eschew DSM-5 in favor of the new system.

RDoC is an ambitious system, but it suffers from its attraction to biological reductionism, giving insufficient weight to environmental effects in disease (Paris and Kirmayer 2016). Thus, it fits the current zeitgeist of psychiatry, but it fails to give adequate priority to gene-environment interactions. RDoC is an attempt to address dissatisfaction with the DSM system in the psychiatric research community by organizing research around specific brain systems. This approach is unlike that used in DSM, in which diagnostic entities are almost entirely based on observable symptoms, self-reports, or behaviors, with the assumption that mental disorders can be grouped into valid and reliable categories based on descriptive phenomenology.

Thirty-five years after DSM-III took this approach to categories of disorder, DSM-5 has still failed to solve the problem of diagnostic reliability, which remains low for most diagnoses, even for common categories such as major depressive disorder (Regier et al. 2013). Moreover, most DSM categories have uncertain validity, and attempts to discover biological markers for disorders have thus far failed (Hyman 2010). Even at the level of genetic associations, much overlap occurs between major categories such as schizophrenia and bipolar disorder (Craddock and Owen 2005). Moreover, DSM categories appear to be highly heterogeneous, and this contributes to high levels of apparent comorbidity (Krueger and Markon 2006). The DSM categories have not been found to be associated with endophenotypes, with specific etiological factors, or with differential responses to specific methods of treatment (Paris 2015a). In spite of decades of research, no findings have emerged to change this verdict.

RDoC hoped to be based on these endophenotypes—that is, the biological basis of psychopathology that DSM failed to deliver. Its developers concluded that the neo-Kraepelinian model and the categories it generates are so flawed that they should be abandoned and that continued reliance on the current diagnostic system can only obstruct progress (Cuthbert and Insel 2013). RDoC is more readily compatible with dimensional diagnoses, in which traits that vary continuously could be more likely to reflect underlying endophenotypes and have stronger relationships to biological measures than categories (Hyman 2010). The concept of dimensional diagnosis was initially attractive to the editors of DSM-5 (Kupfer and Regier 2011), but these proposals foundered. This was due to uncertainty about what kind of dimensional system to apply, to the absence of established cutoff points for psychopathology, and to the absence of strong evidence to justify radical change in the system (Paris 2015a).

Cuthbert and Insel (2013) attributed the failure of research to find convincing explanations for the origins of mental disorders to the fact that diagnoses based on DSM have been a *sine qua non* for the funding and publication of research. Instead, the developers of RDoC looked to neuroscience and cognitive science for models to guide future research. The novelty of RDoC lies in the effort to avoid existing categorical diagnoses of mental disorders, replacing them with a matrix that lists various levels at which researchers can measure processes that may contribute to specific domains of psychopathology. Yet RDoC would still need to develop reliable and valid ways to measure the constructs that characterize each domain and determine their range of variation.

The seven levels or "units of analysis" outlined in RDoC are genes, molecules, cells, circuits, physiology, behavior, and self-reports. Five broad "domains/constructs" were initially proposed (with the assumption that others may be added as they become well established):

1. Negative valence systems (acute threat, potential threat, sustained threat, loss, and frustrative nonreward)
2. Positive valence systems (approach motivation, initial responsiveness to reward, sustained responsiveness to reward, reward learning, and habit)
3. Cognitive systems (attention, perception, working memory, declarative memory, language behavior, and cognitive control)
4. Systems for social processes (affiliation/attachment, social communication, perception/understanding of self, and perception/understanding of others)
5. Arousal/modulatory systems (arousal, biological rhythms, and sleep-wake)

These domains are derived from research in cognitive neuroscience that identifies brain systems governing basic mental functions such as motivation, cognition, emotion, and behavior. Yet although RDoC aims to translate neuroscience into clinically relevant modes and treatment methods, the body of research that RDoC hopes to build on is at an early stage. Moreover, it is hard to see how these five domains alone can account for the great variety of clinical symptoms associated with common mental disorders, such as anxiety or depression, or with severe mental disorders. The current state of research is just not sufficiently mature to account for the complex phenomena that constitute mental illness.

The domains of RDoC also reflect a history of neurobiological research that has explored some systems while leaving others unexplored. As a result, the key domains identified in RDoC have limited correspondence to those derived from other disciplines, including psychology or social psychiatry. RDoC gives special attention to the domain of neural circuitry, based on the importance of networks and connectivity in information processing. This goes along with current attempts to explain behavior and cognition through an understanding of the "connectome," the patterns of neural connectivity within and between specific brain regions. To this end, the NIMH is investing in a Human Connectome Project (Barch 2017). The assumption is that using imaging to detail the functional anatomy of neural networks will yield major advances in understanding the mechanisms behind psychopathology.

RDoC adopts a "bottom up" (rather than "top down") approach, beginning with the assumption that psychiatry is the study and treatment of brain disorders (Insel and Quirion 2005) as opposed to a discipline concerned with disorders of mind, behavior, and inner experience. By defining psychopathology in this way, it institutionalizes neural reductionism. In the past, psychiatry espoused a broader view that included explanation in terms of psychological and interpersonal processes and recognized that research at the levels of mind, behavior, inner experience and social interactions have applications to clinical practice. This multilevel explanatory framework is the basis of the biopsychosocial model (Engel 1980), which promotes a pragmatic and eclectic approach to psychiatric case formulation and treatment. Thus, although it may be very useful if research can identify endophenotypes that underlie mental disorders (Gould and Gottesman 2006), these mechanisms are only clinically meaningful when understood in terms of their interactions with higher levels of mental phenomena that depend on psychological and social processes.

In a commentary on the RDoC system, Parnas (2014) described it as promoting "psychiatry without a psyche." Because of its assumption that psychopathology arises primarily from brain dysfunction, RDoC emphasizes neurobiological levels of explanation (on which five out of seven of the specified levels are based) and downplays psychological and social levels. RDoC therefore breaks with the biopsychosocial model (Engel 1980). Insel and Quirion's (2005) suggestion that psychiatry should redefine itself as the clinical application of neuroscience reflects their assumption that most clinical interventions in psychiatry should be biological rather than psychological. Yet it is known that psychotherapy changes the brain at least as much as pharmacotherapy (Goldapple et al. 2004).

Insel's (2014) description of RDoC as a step toward the fashionable goal of "precision medicine" is an example of how the system is being hyped. "Precision" here refers to tailoring treatment based on specific genetic variations. No evidence has shown that the domains of psychopathology and levels of disability and distress can be linked to specific changes in the genome or to reliable clinical biomarkers. Time may prove RDoC to be "a bridge too far" (Paris and Kirmayer 2016).

In summary, although mental disorders are rooted in underlying traits, their boundaries are fuzzy and unclear. Attempts to address this problem using dimensional scores or concept from neuroscience seem, at least for now, to be simplistic and immature.

PART II

MENTAL DISORDERS

CHAPTER 6

▬ ADHD AND CONDUCT DISORDER

ADHD IS described in DSM-5 (American Psychiatric Association 2013) as a "neurodevelopmental" disorder. This term describes impairments of the growth and development of the brain. However, many major disorders in psychiatry, such as schizophrenia, may be based on similar mechanisms. This term implies a level of knowledge about brain development we do not have.

ADHD cannot be diagnosed unless it begins in childhood. Two general principles govern disorders that begin early in development. The first is that disorders tend to be extreme ends of a continuum of underlying traits. The second is that disorders that then become chronic have a stronger genetic component than those that appear later in life. ADHD is an example, and its heritability in behavior genetic research, confirmed by twin and adoption studies, has been estimated at 74% (Faraone and Larsson 2019). ADHD was one of the disorders studied by the Psychiatric Genome-Wide Association Study Consortium (Sullivan 2010).

We need to examine the boundaries of ADHD. This is a disorder that overlaps with many other categories and may be undergoing a diagnostic epidemic (Paris 2015b).

BOUNDARIES OF ADHD

ADHD has uncertain boundaries. This condition may not even be viewed as a category but might better be conceptualized as a continuously varying dimension (Faraone and Larsson 2019). When a diagnosis has fuzzy edges, it is tempting to extend its scope. This has happened with other categories, such as bipolar disorder (Paris 2012). Judging by the rapid increase of stimulant prescriptions in the last few decades (Olfson et al. 2013), ADHD diagnosis has become much more frequent in clinical practice. The real reason for broadening the ADHD diagnosis is the success of stimulants in treating some of these patients. Clinicians tend to favor the diagnosis of conditions that have a specific pharmacological treatment.

No validated test can identify ADHD with sensitivity and specificity. Checklists such as the Conners Comprehensive Behavior Rating Scales (Conners 2008) have been widely used, but the long version, which takes 90 minutes to complete, is not suitable for a busy practice. A shorter version, the Conners Clinical Index, has only 25 questions and can be filled out either by patients, parents, or teachers. Yet these scales still fail to draw a well-validated boundary around ADHD, making make it difficult to interpret data about the prevalence of this disorder. Even Keith Conners, prior to his death, was deeply concerned about the problem of overdiagnosis (Frances and Carroll 2017).

Estimates of ADHD prevalence vary when definitions are unclear. At the higher end, it has been claimed to be between 5% and 10% in boys and between 2% and 4% in girls (Barkley 2014). Another set of authorities estimate overall prevalence is about 5% (Faraone et al. 2003). A third and more conservative estimate based on a World Health Organization survey suggests 1.4%–3% (Thapar and Cooper 2016). Even the lowest prevalence estimates are higher than those for many psychiatric disorders. The most likely explanation is that we are looking not at a narrowly defined category but at a widely distributed trait.

Two components in the construct of ADHD are defined in DSM-5: 1) a deficit in maintaining attention, and 2) an abnormal level of activity and impulsivity. Different patients can have a predominance of one or the other. Increased activity associated with impulsivity is most likely to bring children to clinical attention and is the most disabling aspect of the condition. Because boys are usually more physically active than girls, ADHD with hyperactivity is more common in males, whereas ADHD without hyperactivity has a relatively equal sex distribution (Hechtman 2016). ADHD with hyperactivity is highly comorbid with other diagnoses, particularly conduct disorder (Spencer 2006). The combination of both diagnoses is what most often leads to the referral of children for assessment (Thapar and Cooper 2016). When ADHD is not accompanied by conduct disorder, as is more often the case among girls, it may not be identified unless it leads to problems with academic performance.

Although ADHD begins in childhood, it does not always "burn out" over time. Follow-up studies show that about a half of cases continue to have symptoms in adulthood and that at least one-fifth and up to one-third of cases, particularly those with comorbid conduct disorder, will develop antisocial personality disorder (Barkley 2014; Hechtman 2016). These findings have sparked interest in diagnosing and treating previously unrecognized cases in adult populations. However, overdiagnosis of ADHD in adults is a real danger (Paris et al. 2015) because, among other reasons, clinicians can diagnose patients who do not have an established history of childhood ADHD as required by DSM-5. Another reason is that adults can have attention problems with other origins (e.g., depression, anxiety). When ADHD is overdiagnosed, stimulants may be used, much as psychiatrists in the 1950s prescribed amphetamine to increase energy or focus.

In DSM-5, ADHD is required to begin in childhood, not later than age 12 years. (The age at onset was extended from previous editions of the manual, which required symptoms to begin by age 6.) How can one be sure about a history many years later? Some patients claim to have a self-diagnosis of ADHD or to have been formally "diagnosed," usually on the basis of a quick clinical assessment or a checklist. Sometimes the argument is made that ADHD must have been present in childhood but never identified—a difficult position to sustain given the wide variation in attention and hyperactivity among normally developing children.

An important paper by Moffitt et al. (2015) examined ADHD symptoms among adult participants in the Dunedin birth cohort study, allowing researchers direct access to childhood problems uninfluenced by the vagaries of human memory. The main finding was that very few individuals whose symptoms seemed to meet criteria for the diagnosis as adults had ever had the same problems as children. The authors therefore wondered if the childhood-onset and adult-onset symptoms reflect entirely different diagnostic entities. If so, then many, if not most, cases of adult ADHD could be misdiagnosed.

The more familial a case of ADHD, the earlier is its onset and the more likely it is to continue into adulthood (Biederman et al. 1996). This raises the question as to whether it was wise to change the threshold in DSM-5 for age at onset (from 6 to 12 years). We also do not know how to determine clinically significant cutoff points in attention, hyperactivity, and impulsivity. Finally, we do know how separate ADHD is from the other diagnoses with which it is comorbid.

GENETIC PREDISPOSITIONS

Faraone and Larsson (2019) reviewed evidence showing that ADHD is highly heritable. Symptom counts based on parent and teacher reports can give heritability estimates ranging from 77% to 88%. However, they also noted that self-report measures, both in adolescents and adults, give much lower estimates of around 30%. (This discrepancy could reflect lack of patient insight but merits further investigation.) No biomarkers for ADHD are known. Meta-analyses find a replicated statistical relationship between ADHD dopamine system genes such as *DRD4* (Li et al. 2006). However, there is a missing heritability, and this gene explains only a small part of the variance.

A meta-analysis of genome-wide association studies (GWASs) identified 12 loci associated with ADHD but again pointed to a combination of many common polymorphisms. Polygenic risk scores point to an overlap between ADHD and other major mental disorders such as schizophrenia (Hamshere et al. 2013). The polygenic risk score was also much higher in those who also had conduct disorder. Much has been written about the role of dopamine and the *DRD4* gene in ADHD, but Thapar and Cooper (2016) pointed out that *DRD4* and other genes are more related to conduct disorder than to the core syndrome of ADHD. Perhaps what is inherited is not ADHD itself but traits that predispose to this disorder and to comorbid disorders. The last word is not in, but a very-large-scale GWAS found 12 genes linked to ADHD, accounting for 22% of the variance (Demontis et al. 2019). The genetic risk is indeed related to impulsivity and inattention but also overlaps with the risk for depression, obesity, and diabetes.

In clinical work, because we lack biomarkers for ADHD, we are stuck with checklists. A meta-analysis of functional MRI studies, including both children and adults (Cortese et al. 2012), examining areas associated with executive function found abnormalities related to the clinical symptoms of the disorder (reduced attention and executive functions). However, these findings are by no means specific to the disorder. We are not in a position to diagnose ADHD (or any mental disorder) with a brain scan.

ENVIRONMENTAL STRESSORS

ADHD is also associated with psychosocial risk factors. This was best shown in a Danish birth cohort study that predicted the disorder by the presence of a set of standard indicators of adversity from infancy on (Ostergaard et al. 2016). The risks are low social class, severe marital discord, large family size, paternal criminality, maternal mental disorder, and placement in out-of-home care. None are specific to ADHD; they are the general risk factors for psychopathology in children, identified in a classic epidemiological study (Rutter et al. 1976).

These measures of adversity, in concert, significantly raise the risk for the development of any psychiatric diagnosis in children. Scores on a scale measuring all these factors are better predictors than was any single factor of the development of psychiatric disorders of all types. By and large, environmental factors depend on cumulative effects of multiple risks. Biederman et al. (1995) also used Rutter's scale to assess the environmental risk factors for ADHD. Again, the more indicators present, the more likely children were to develop the disorder. Yet the same risk factors predicted the development of other "externalizing" disorders, as well as "internalizing" disorders, such as depression and anxiety.

GENE-ENVIRONMENT INTERACTIONS

Attentional capacity and activity-impulsivity levels are intercorrelated and continuously distributed in the population. At some threshold, these traits can become problematic. This threshold is influenced by the strength of predispositions and on the number of stressors. One study attempted to examine interactions between genes and environment (Grizenko et al. 2012). It found that children whose mothers who were stressed during pregnancy and who also had a polymorphism in *DRD4* were more likely to develop ADHD. However, only a small percentage of the variance was accounted for.

To put the problem in a wider perspective, ADHD derives from a widely distributed set of traits that need not, in and of itself, be dysfunctional. Thus, every trait has to be understood in terms of its original function in what evolutionary psychologists call the "environment of evolutionary adaptiveness." In prehistorical societies, men with a shorter attention span and higher levels of activity-impulsivity might have actually functioned better in settings where overt aggression and rapid responses were useful for survival. However, in a modern society, interactions occur between these traits and specific social demands. One is the expectation for young boys to sit down and pay attention in a classroom. Sitting quietly, listening to a teacher, or reading a book has no biological advantage. Rather, these sociocultural expectations have only developed in modern societies. As recently as a few generations ago, children who could not cope would leave school at an early age and go out to work. ADHD was first described in the medical literature about 100 years ago (Still 1902), at the same time child labor was being abolished.

Children with ADHD are a heterogeneous population. Many have strong biological predispositions associated with an early onset and a chronic course of illness. Others have weaker predispositions that only become amplified to dysfunctional levels when exposed to major environmental stressors. Faraone and Larsson (2019) summarized the issues as follows:

> Accumulating evidence from family, twin, and molecular genetic studies suggests that the disorder we know as ADHD is the extreme of a dimensional trait in the population. The dimensional nature of ADHD has wide-ranging implications. If we view ADHD as analogous to cholesterol levels, then diagnostic approaches should focus on defining the full continuum of "ADHD-traits" along with clinically meaningful thresholds for defining who does and does not need treatment and who has clinically subthreshold traits that call for careful monitoring. The dimensional nature of ADHD should also shift the debate about the increases in ADHD's prevalence in recent years. Instead of assuming that misdiagnoses are the main explanation for the increased prevalence, perhaps researchers should explore to what extent the threshold for diagnosis has decreased over time and whether changes in the threshold are clinically sensible or not. (p. 570)

CONDUCT DISORDER

Conduct disorder is a highly prevalent disorder in children. affecting 9.5% of children (males 12.0%, females 7.1%) (Nock et al. 2006). Like ADHD, conduct disorder begins in childhood but is associated with later adult disorders. One-third of children with conduct disorder seen in clinical settings go on to develop antisocial personality disorder; outcome is more likely when more symptoms are present, when symptoms are severe, and when they have an early onset (Zoccolillo et al. 1992). Moreover, conduct disorder can also be a precursor of other forms of psychopathology ranging from mood disorder to psychosis.

Conduct disorder, in contrast to ADHD, is moderately heritable, at the level of 50% (Salvatore and Dick 2018). It is one of the few mental disorders that shows significant variance (14%) related to shared environment (Polderman et al. 2015). Using multiple informants, a large-scale twin study in Wales (Scourfield et al. 2004) found even larger unshared environmental effects from parental reports (30%–40%), with a genetic risk of about 40%.

As discussed in Chapter 4, there is conflicting evidence about the extent to which genes affecting monoamine oxidase are implicated in antisocial behavior. GWASs have been inconclusive (Dick et al. 2011). Conduct disorder is best understood in terms of gene-environment interactions (Dodge 2009). Cadoret et al. (1995) showed that even when adoptees have a biological parent with antisocial personality disorder, they only develop symptoms if they also experience an adverse adoptive home environment.

We also need to define subpopulations with conduct disorder more precisely to take heterogeneity into account. For example, in the Dunedin sample, Moffitt et al. (2001) reported that early-onset conduct disorder was more likely to go on to antisocial behavior and that when symptoms begin in adolescence, they usually remit by young adulthood. The temperamental differences that lead to antisocial behavior can be observed as early as age 3, as shown in the Dunedin study (Caspi et al. 1996). Kagan (1994) noted that "behaviorally inhibited" (i.e., abnormally anxious and shy) children never develop these symptoms.

The environmental predictors of conduct disorder are essentially those described by Rutter et al. (1976) as adversities leading to most forms of psychopathology in children. Yet children who go on to develop adult antisocial behavior are a genetically different group from those who do not. The subgroup of children who go on to develop antisocial personality have stronger predispositions. Genetic factors seem to be weaker in adolescent delinquency, when factors such as joining a gang play a larger role. Instead, these children are responding to a stressful environment from which they can eventually escape. In summary, research findings are consistent with the following model:

1. Children with conduct disorder are heterogeneous, with most having no specific genetic liability and with symptoms being precipitated primarily by family dysfunction.
2. Genetic factors are more important in those with early and more severe symptoms and in those who go on to develop antisocial personality disorder.
3. Even when genetic factors predispose to conduct disorder, these effects only emerge in the presence of interactions with family pathology.

CHAPTER 7

▬ SCHIZOPHRENIA

GENETIC RISK FACTORS

We have known for decades that schizophrenia has a strong genetic pre-disposition (Coelewij and Curtis 2018). The success of pharmacological treatment and the relative failure of psychotherapy to manage acute symptoms are in accord with a biologically based etiology. A meta-analysis of twin studies estimated the genetic liability to schizophrenia at 81% (Sullivan et al. 2003). The heritability of the disorder is even greater when one takes into account that the first-degree relatives of probands can have spectrum disorders such as schizotypal personality (Sullivan 2005). Adoption studies of schizophrenia show that if an adopted child has a biological parent with this form of pathology, risk for the disorder greatly increases (Leo 2006)

Studies of high-risk children support the same conclusions. Cohorts of offspring of mothers with schizophrenia have been followed for about 25 years and have been shown to be at risk for both schizophrenia and schizophrenia spectrum disorders (Erlenmeyer-Kimling et al. 1995). Moreover, these children, even during childhood, show "soft neurological signs" similar to those seen in adult patients with schizophrenia (Walker et al. 1994). Research has, however, failed to identify any specific biological marker associated with a diathesis to schizophrenia. The most consistent markers in the research literature are abnormal eye movements, which are also found in those with schizotypal personality (Levy et al. 2004).

Yet in spite of massive research efforts over several decades, the precise biological nature of the genetic predisposition to schizophrenia remains unknown. Genome-wide association studies have shown that hundreds of common polymorphisms seem to be involved (Bergen and Petryshen 2012; Coelewij and Curtis 2018). A polygenic risk score (PRS) can help define liability but does not usefully predict emergence of the full disorder (Riglin et al. 2017). However, some have suggested that because schizophrenia carries a large genetic load, PRS might be used in this way (Binder 2019; Kalin 2019). This conclusion is supported by the fact that PRS accounts for more liability on schizophrenia than in other mental disorders (Zheutlin et al. 2019).

In contrast, a meta-analysis found that no "historical" candidate genes are associated with the diagnosis (Johnson et al. 2017). As discussed in Chapter 2, some research has suggested that one deletion site (q22.11) is related to schizophrenia but is present only in a small minority of cases Another problem is that we remain unsure about whether schizophrenia is one disease or many, or whether it can be separated from other psychoses. The same genes can increase vulnerability for schizophrenia and for bipolar mood disorder (Craddock et al. 2006; Cross-Disorder Group of the Psychiatric Genomics Consortium 2019).

Schizophrenia is more severe in men than in women (Canuso and Pandina 2007). Milder forms of schizophrenia and schizophrenia spectrum disorders probably derive from a less severe genetic loading, whereas an early onset of illness is also associated with higher genetic loading (Gottesman 1991). We do not know the mechanisms by which genetic variations affect brain function in schizophrenia. One suggestion is that problems arise during synaptic pruning in adolescence (in which a large number of neurons are removed), but the evidence for this hypothesis remains unclear (Boksa 2012). One of the most popular theories was based on the fact that pharmacological agents block different types of dopamine receptors, suggesting abnormalities in dopaminergic transmission in schizophrenia (Seeman et al. 1997). However, even after decades of research, the model remains controversial (Moncrieff 2009).

Given the complexity of this disorder, it may not be readily reduced to the action of a single neurotransmitter and its receptors. It could be more useful to look at markers for abnormal neuroconnectivity (Millan et al. 2016). Neuropsychological abnormalities are found with some consistency in patients with schizophrenia. A number of observations, including abnormal eye tracking and an aberrant P300 response on electroencephalography, suggest a particular difficulty in integrating complex stimuli (Bilder 1996). Decreases in frontal lobe activation have been visualized using imaging methods in patients with schizophrenia, although similar findings have been reported in bipolar disorder (Birur et al. 2017).

Negative symptoms in schizophrenia may derive from different mechanisms than positive symptoms. The deficit symptoms of the disease might be better markers of a genetic predisposition and may be accompanied by ventricular enlargement (Gottesman 1991). Genetic factors may also influence neural development, most particularly the migration of neurons during fetal life (Weinberger 1987). It is also possible that negative symptoms, particularly those associated with objective evidence of brain damage, reflect effects of the environmental factors in schizophrenia, such as viral infections during fetal or perinatal life. Brain damage may also be responsible for cognitive deficits in schizophrenia that appear well before the onset of the disease. These changes would be associated with cognitive abnormalities that are developmental, deriving from connections between brain areas. Many of these connections develop during fetal life, whereas others occur across development. Because synaptic pruning is not complete until early adulthood, this might help explain the age at onset of the disorder.

One other environmental trigger has a specific effect on people at genetic risk for schizophrenia. This is cannabis, which has is a dose-response relationship (Colizzi and Murray 2018); cannabis use and heavy use of synthetics further raise the risk for the illness. This situation runs parallel to the triggering of lung cancer in susceptible individuals by heavy smoking.

ENVIRONMENTAL RISK FACTORS

Environmental risk factors have a place in schizophrenia: in a meta-analysis, shared environmental effects were estimated to be 11% (Sullivan et al. 2003). Moreover, heritability studies show that half of monozygotic twins are discordant for schizophrenia (Gottesman 1991). To some extent, these findings reflect differences in the severity of the disorder, because unaffected twins are more likely to have traits in the "schizophrenia spectrum." When the full spectrum is taken into account, even stronger patterns of heritability are found (Kendler et al. 1993a). In a classical and still fascinating study of identical quadruplets with schizophrenia (Rosenthal 1963), severity of illness ranged from a single episode of positive symptoms to a chronic course with negative symptoms. The question is what these environmental factors might be. Are they biological, or psychosocial, or both? A predisposition to schizophrenia can be activated by various factors that lead to brain injury. In this view, the genetic predisposition increases sensitivity to these risk factors, but effects on the brain act as the trigger, unleashing a process that uncovers the illness.

It has long been believed that problems in family life or in child development have little relationship to schizophrenia; however, research has challenged this point of view (Morgan and Gayer-Anderson 2016). A relationship with child abuse or trauma has been documented, and this finding has been replicated (Sideli et al. 2012). Actually, child maltreatment is a risk factor for many mental disorders, and specific types of psychopathology that emerge are determined by genetic predispositions. Critics of psychiatry, such as Bentall (2009), have used these findings to question purely biological models. It makes more sense to understand that schizophrenia, however strong the genetics, requires a biopsychosocial model.

Some psychological factors in the family environment could affect remission and the ultimate outcome of the disorder. A large body of research has described "expressed emotion"—that is, affectively charged criticism from relatives—influences the rate of relapse in schizophrenia (Falloon et al. 1984). However, these responses may also reflect understandable frustration among family members (Hooley 2007).

Social factors may also play a role in the etiology of schizophrenia. There is a similar prevalence rate of the disorder over the globe (Jablensky et al. 1992), but schizophrenia is more episodic and less chronic in traditional societies (Leff 1988). One possible explanation is that the stronger family and community supports in traditional societies act as protective factors. Even within North America, the Vermont Longitudinal Study (Harding et al. 1987) found many cases in which patients living in rural areas remained functional for long periods.

In modern societies, where schizophrenia leads to more severe dysfunction, the fertility of affected individuals is low. However, patients with schizophrenia spectrum disorders could be more likely to reproduce in traditional societies, where identity and social roles are prescribed rather than discovered. Meehl (1990) hypothesized that for every case of overt schizophrenia, there could be many others in which "schizotaxic" traits are present without causing psychosis.

In the past few decades, evidence has accumulated that immigration can be an important risk factor for schizophrenia. In research led by the British psychiatrist Robin Murray, it was found that West Indian migrants to the United Kingdom had a much higher frequency of the disorder than those who remained at home (Morgan et al. 2010). This relationship is explained by the concept of "social defeat," the idea that when migrants fail to find a place in the new society, they are more subject to severe mental illness (Cantor-Graae and Selten 2005). These findings, first described in the United Kingdom, have been replicated in other societies in which migrants from developing countries struggled to find a place. However, these relationships are not universal: some migrants seem to be more vulnerable than others (Morgan et al. 2019).

It is also worth noting that environmental risks that interfere with prenatal development can be associated with an outcome of schizophrenia. This relationship has been observed in studies of children born around the time of the Dutch famine of 1944–45 (Hoek et al. 1998).

GENE-ENVIRONMENT INTERACTIONS

Although schizophrenia is mainly biological, it is also biopsychosocial in origin. A large-scale European study (Guloksuz et al. 2019) concluded:

> Evidence was found for additive interaction of molecular genetic risk state for schizophrenia....with the presence of lifetime regular cannabis use and exposure to early-life adversities (sexual abuse, emotional abuse, emotional neglect, and bullying), but not with the presence of hearing impairment, season of birth (winter birth), and exposure to physical abuse or physical neglect in childhood....Our results suggest that the etiopathogenesis of schizophrenia involves genetic underpinnings that act by making individuals more sensitive to the effects of some environmental exposures. (p. 182)

Thus, the following conclusions are in accord with our present knowledge:

1. Schizophrenia does not develop without a specific genetic predisposition.
2. This predisposition may express itself as full-blown illness or as disorders in the "schizophrenia spectrum."
3. The predisposition is more likely to lead to illness in the presence of additional stressors, which can be biological, psychological, or social.

A BRIEF NOTE ON BIPOLAR DISORDERS

The heritability of bipolarity appears to be similar to that of schizophrenia (Kieseppä et al. 2004), and a fair degree of genetic overlap occurs between these disorders (Lichtenstein et al. 2009). Some have gone so far as to deny the validity of the Kraepelinian dichotomy separating them (Craddock and Owen 2005).

There is less research on the role of factors in bipolar disorders than in schizophrenia. In a review, Paykel (2003) noted that environmental stressors tend to be most associated with the first episode. In a longitudinal study of adolescents, Pan et al. (2017) found that stressful life events were unusually common, both in those who had parents with bipolar disorder and those who did not. It may well be that environmental factors can be triggers for manic episodes. However, these relationships have not been widely documented, and there is less research on the role of psychosocial factors in bipolar disorders than in schizophrenia.

CHAPTER 8

— DEPRESSIVE DISORDERS

THE BOUNDARIES OF DEPRESSIVE ILLNESS

Depressed mood is a familiar experience for most of us. Mild symptoms reflecting lowered mood after a loss or disappointment are all but universal. Yet there is no clear cutoff point on the continuum between normal sadness and incapacitating depression. Depression as a disorder has been hypothesized to be a biologically patterned response that has an adaptive function: accepting defeat or evoking help from others (Nesse 2019). Severe stressors may produce depression in virtually anyone, but in those who are predisposed to depression, symptoms can appear with only mild environmental provocation.

The boundaries of major depression have long been a problem for psychiatry (Parker et al. 2017). An important unanswered question is whether depression is *one* disease with various levels of severity or *many* diseases, each with a different casual pathway. We do not even know whether unipolar and bipolar depressions are different illnesses or represent different forms of the same illness. We also do not know whether melancholic and nonmelancholic or psychotic and nonpsychotic depressions are unique disorders or more severe aspects of the same illness. Moreover, depression overlaps with a number of other psychiatric diagnoses with which it tends to be "comorbid." Genetic epidemiological studies suggest that the genetic and environmental factors for depression are not specific but overlap with those for anxiety disorders, eating disorders, substance use disorders, and personality disorders (Kendler et al. 2007).

Over the past 150 years, mood disorders have been classified in different ways (Berrios 1992). DSM-5 emphasizes the differences between unipolar and bipolar disorders, between melancholic and nonmelancholic depression, and between psychotic or nonpsychotic depression (American Psychiatric Association 2013). Major depressive disorder (MDD) is one of the most common disorders in the community and is more frequent in women, with a lifetime prevalence of 21%, than in men (3%) (Kessler et al. 1993).

To make a diagnosis of MDD according to DSM criteria requires, in addition to a depressed mood, the presence of five of nine specific criteria associated with depression, which must be present for at least 2 weeks. This definition might be recited from memory by psychiatrists. It has the advantage of being reasonably precise and practically useful. The problem is that clinicians have come to *reify* this construct. The diagnosis of MDD is a barrier to understanding the many factors that contribute to clinical phenomena. We need not think of depression as a unitary disorder.

Parker et al. (2017) argued that DSM makes a mistake by considering all depressions to be one illness with different levels of severity. They see at least two separate disorders, the *melancholic* type (which responds best to drugs and electroconvulsive therapy) and the *nonmelancholic* type (milder depressions that constitute the majority of cases in practice but respond less consistently to drugs). The limitations of the MDD construct are also shown by the fact that a number of permutations of symptoms can yield the same diagnosis. There are nine criteria, and although the patient must have either depressed mood or a loss of interest and pleasure, it is sufficient to have five of the others. This means the diagnostic criteria can be met in multiple ways. This bar is also very low, especially the requirement for a duration of only 2 weeks. I wonder how many of us have not experienced depressive symptoms for this long after a major loss.

Clinicians all too often assume that making a diagnosis of MDD is a reasonable basis for a decision as to whether to prescribe antidepressants. Many are not even put off by comorbidities that point in a different direction, such as the finding that patients who also have a personality disorder do not usually respond to medication (Newton-Jones et al. 2006). Moreover, DSM was never intended to be a treatment guide, nor did it ever claim that its diagnoses are a guide to any form of therapy. Yet that is how clinicians often use it.

Not many realize that the diagnosis of MDD is, as shown in the DSM-5 field trials (Regier et al. 2013), not all that reliable in practice because it has no sharp boundary. Depression, even more than schizophrenia, is a *spectrum* disorder. This means that the predisposition to become depressed varies in intensity, and its expression depends on environmental factors. At one end of the spectrum lies incapacitating illness, such as recurrent unipolar depression with melancholic or psychotic features, whereas at the other end is persistent depressive disorder (formerly called dysthymia), in which one may only observe a chronic but nonsevere lowering of mood. The majority of cases take an intermediate form.

The depressive spectrum is not smooth and continuous. We can find peaks and valleys representing qualitatively different forms of illness. For this reason, there could be multiple thresholds for depression, each reflecting different forms of illness. Thus, melancholic and nonmelancholic depressions could have a different weighting of risk factors, with predispositions playing a stronger role in the melancholic type and stressors playing a greater role in the nonmelancholic type. This crucial distinction is lost by considering depression to be *one* thing. Given the low bar for diagnosis used today (symptoms lasting only 2 weeks), it is hard to believe that all depressions are variants of the same pathological process.

A good deal of empirical evidence supports this view. The more severe the depression, the more likely it is to find a positive family history, and twin studies show double the concordance in recurrent unipolar illness than in unipolar patients with fewer than three episodes (Nurnberger and Gershon 1992). Recent negative life events are more likely to be found in nonendogenous patients (Brown et al. 1994).

GENETIC PREDISPOSITIONS FOR DEPRESSION

There can be little doubt that a vulnerability to depression is inherited. A meta-analysis of twin research data shows that the heritability rate for depression is 37%, that data from family studies show a two- to threefold increase in the risk of depression in first-degree offspring of patients with depression, that an early onset is associated with higher heritability, and that severe forms of depression are more heritable (Sullivan et al. 2000). Other behavioral genetic studies have consistently shown that depressive disorders are heritable. In a large-scale twin study in Sweden (Kendler et al. 2018), the heritability was 41%. However, if less severe forms of depression are less heritable, we should hesitate to generalize about a category that is heterogeneous. In spite of all these problems, many researchers (e.g., Corfield et al. 2017) consider depression to lie on a spectrum and suggest that what might be called "minor depression" is only a variant of the major type. Perhaps they are influenced by the practice of prescribing antidepressants to patients with any kind of depression in spite of any comorbid diagnosis.

One consistent finding in the literature is that severe depression is more heritable than mild depression. Kendler et al. (1992a) found that the presence of vegetative symptoms is linked with increased heritability. Genetic factors are also stronger in depressions that lead to hospitalization (McGuffin et al. 1991, 1996). Kendler et al. (1996) concluded that different mechanisms are involved in depressive illness of differing levels of severity. Persistent depressive disorder is a condition in which symptoms are milder but chronic and responds less predictably to antidepressant therapy than does MDD (Kocsis et al. 1991). Cases of persistent depressive disorder that begin in adolescence are often associated with personality disorders (Pepper et al. 1995). This raises a question: when does chronic depression distort personality, and when does personality pathology cause chronic depression?

The comorbidity of any form of depression with a personality disorder predicts chronicity (Alnaes and Torgersen 1997). It is also interesting to note that persistent depressive disorder has a comorbidity of 60% with personality disorders, three to four times greater than that of major depression (Pepper et al. 1995). Moreover, when depression or dysthymia have an early onset, they are strongly comorbid with personality disorders, particularly those in Cluster B (Fava et al. 1996; Riso et al. 1996).

In the mildest forms of depression, predispositions may be expressed not as overt illness but as personality traits. A large body of research (Coyne and Whiffen 1995) points to two personality traits that increase the likelihood that environmental stressors will lead to depressive illness. The first is called "sociotropic" or "dependent," a construct describing individuals who are unusually sensitive to loss or abandonment. The second is called "autonomous" or "self-critical," a construct describing individuals who are unusually sensitive to failure to achieve their goals. Like other traits, these personality characteristics are themselves genetically influenced, as shown by their correlations with broader personality dimensions, such as neuroticism (Coyne and Whiffen 1995).

In summary, depression is heterogeneous. Some cases show a strong genetic component, whereas others demonstrate stronger environmental influence. In the future, we may have clear-cut biological markers to identify the predisposition to mood disorders. These might help us develop better ways of subtyping mood disorders, thereby increasing our ability to disentangle the effects of nature and nurture. We are still very far from being able to estimate the effects of specific polymorphisms on the risk for depression. Some had hoped to find genes associated with monoamines, but this has never been confirmed. Genome-wide association studies on MDD (Power et al. 2017; Wray et al. 2018) have identified only a few polymorphisms strongly associated with the disorder, none of which accounts for much of the variance. Of particular interest, a recent meta-analysis confirmed this result and, contrary to earlier received opinion, failed to find any link between depression and the serotonin transporter gene (Border et al. 2019). A review article summarized this literature as follows:

> Family and twin studies have demonstrated that the contribution of genetic factors to the risk of the onset of DDs [depressive disorders] is quite large. Various methodological approaches (analysis of candidate genes, genome-wide association analysis, genome-wide sequencing) have been used, and a large number of the associations between genes and different clinical DD variants and DD subphenotypes have been published. However, in most cases, these associations have not been confirmed in replication studies, and only a small number of genes have been proven to be associated with DD development risk. (Shadrina et al. 2018, p. 334)

ROLE OF STRESSORS IN DEPRESSION

Gene-environment models help us avoid the fruitless debates so common in the past as to whether depressions are "endogenous" or "reactive." They can be, and usually are, both. There need not be *specific* stressors associated with the onset of mood disorders. Risk factors can derive from interpersonal loss, work problems, or physical illness. Research demonstrates increases in the number of life events prior to the onset of affective episodes (Paykel 1992). Chronic stress is also a risk factor (Hammen et al. 2005). It is well established that stressful events affect the brain through the hypothalamic-pituitary axis, but many other pathways can be involved (Yang et al. 2015).

The main psychological stressor thought to lead to depression is interpersonal loss (Bowlby 1980). Psychiatrists have long assumed that pathological grief is an important cause of clinical depression. However, they may be mistaken in attributing simple cause and effect to this sequence of events. For every case in which depression follows grief, in many others it does not. The empirical evidence that recent losses increase the risk for depressive episodes has been surprisingly weak (Paykel 1992).

However, some evidence has shown that early losses can sensitize people with recent losses (Slavich et al. 2011).

DSM-5 chose to drop a grief exclusion in making a diagnosis of MDD. The rationale was that although transient symptoms are common, only some people develop a major depression after a loss. This decision has been criticized for medicalizing normal sadness (Horwitz and Wakefield 2007). Others have suggested that we should go the other way and consider other major stressors as exclusions (Nesse 2019). Still others have pointed out that patients with grief can also benefit from treatment for depression (Zisook and Kendler 2007). Wakefield et al. (2017) argued that "uncomplicated" depression is a normal variant that is not, unlike melancholic or severe depression, notably associated with suicide. As they concluded:

> The overpathologization of depression can only be addressed by focusing on the distinction between normal distress and indicators of dysfunctional psychological functioning. The criteria for uncomplicated depression are one empirically supported attempt to distinguish between depressive disorder and distress that meets the criteria for major depression. This distinction should not be the only, or final, attempt at distinguishing pathological versus non-pathological cases of MDD. However, the strength and consistency of the research findings suggest that uncomplicated depression is one category of false positives and confirm the belief that the category of MDD requires rethinking in light of evolutionary considerations. If we take people as they are rather than as we would prefer that they be, then painful as it may be uncomplicated depression is a normal-range, not disordered, emotional reaction, and informed consent and treatment strategies should be sensitive to this reality. (p. 65)

At this point, the idea that losses early in life are a risk factor for depression later in life remains controversial. Decades ago, Brown and Harris (1978), in a widely quoted study, found that the early loss of a mother was an important risk factor for depression in women. However, many other scenarios could be relevant. Parker (1983) found that depressed patients consistently report that their parents were both neglectful and overcontrolling, a pattern he termed "affectionless control." Rutter (1989) concluded that of all possible childhood adversities, a consistent lack of affection in childhood is the most consistent risk factor for nonmelancholic adult depression. Keep in mind that all these findings were based on retrospective perceptions of currently depressed patients, who are more likely to see the past in a negative light. To be considered as etiological factors in depression, children who experience parental neglect would have to be prospectively followed into adulthood to see if they develop mood disorders. This relationship has thus far been confirmed in the cohort followed by the Children in the Community Study (Cohen et al. 2017).

In the case of childhood losses, we lack consistent evidence demonstrating an increase the risk for adult depression: the association has been either not replicated or shown to be less important than other risks. For example, in a large-scale twin study, Kendler et al. (1991b) found that loss of a parent prior to age 17 years explained very little of the variance in the development of MDD. Slavich et al. (2011) contested that verdict, presenting evidence that early adversity is associated with a lower threshold of reactivity to life stressors later in life. In this view, the main explanation for the contradiction is that this kind of risk affects different people differently, depending on genetic predispositions. Another issue could be that depression is not one thing. If depression describes many different disorders, that could explain all kinds of problems with research and would also account for contradictory evidence about the efficacy of treatment for MDD. By and large, it seems reasonable to conclude that the importance of recent and remote life events in the etiology of mood disorders has been exaggerated. The more general principle is that negative events have different effects on predisposed individuals.

Although bipolar illness affects men and women equally, unipolar depression is about twice as common in females (Weissman and Klerman 1985). Is this a genetic difference, an environmental difference or both? One possibility is that sex differences are an artefact, because women are more likely to talk about their feelings whereas men are more likely to deny them or drown their sorrows in drink. A classic study of the Amish (Egeland and Hostetter 1983), in whom substance abuse is quite rare, found an equal prevalence for depression in men and women. Nonetheless, Weissman and Klerman (1985) concluded that sex differences in depression have been observed in many countries around the world and are probably real.

We know of no sex-linked genetic factors determining the threshold for depressive illness. Nevertheless, in view of the well-known effects of hormones on mood, it seems likely that these fluctuations could be one factor making women more vulnerable to depression. Another possibility is that prevalence may be attributed to some degree by psychosocial factors that differentially effect males and females. For example, one of the most important correlates of depression in women is an unhappy marriage (Klerman and Weissman 1989). These effects may be less strong if women have other sources of self-esteem. One early epidemiological study (Srole and Fischer 1980) found that as women entered the work force, their mental health improved.

One of the most striking research findings concerning depression is the increase in its prevalence over recent decades. This *cohort effect* was established in American samples (Robins and Regier 1991) and has been observed in other countries (Klerman and Weissman 1989). However, more recent studies have found that the prevalence of MDD is now much more stable both in adults (Wang et al. 2017) and in children and adolescents (Costello et al. 2006). Yet the increase in prevalence observed in the latter part of the past century requires an explanation. It is possible that MDD is more likely to be recognized now than in the past. Another line of argument could be derived from social factors. Rapid cohort changes in stressors over a single generation could reflect *social change*. The most likely candidates would be increased rates of family breakdown or a breakdown in community structures outside the family, leading to compromised social networks (Rutter and Smith 1995). The effects of social stressors would still, however, be mediated by gene-environment interactions.

Moreover, depression may be a universal phenomenon that expressed itself differently in symptoms depending on culture, either in physical or in psychological complaints (Murphy 1982). In a population-based survey conducted in 10 countries (Ferrari et al. 2013), the global burden of disease for MDD was indeed global, although the burden was higher in the Middle East. Depression had similar symptoms, age at onset, and sex distribution in all the countries studied.

GENE-ENVIRONMENT INTERACTIONS IN DEPRESSION

Without a genetic diathesis, negative life experiences and difficult interpersonal relations need not cause depressive illness. Without environmental stressors, the predisposition to depression may never become activated. In a large-scale community study of adult female twins, Kendler et al. (2006) examined the genetic and environmental factors in individuals with unipolar depression. The best-fitting model, which predicted about half of the variance in liability to MDD, was derived from interactions between a heritable component and the influence of psychosocial stressors.

Gene-environment interactions make any model of the causes of depression more complex. Stressful life events are only weak predictors of mood disorders and may even reflect indirect genetic influences, because those who are predisposed to depression are more likely to experience negative events. For example, those who become easily depressed are also more likely to have difficulties with their interpersonal relationships. Individuals prone to depression may have specific personality traits, termed *neuroticism*—that is, high levels of pessimism and worry that actually make negative life events more likely (Kendler et al. 1993b). Psychological research finds that pessimists are often more realistic about life's challenges (Lewinsohn et al. 1980), but pessimism can also bring on negative life events through a mechanism of "self-fulfilling prophecy."

Depression is a more chronic illness than was previously believed. One likely explanation involves a "kindling" theory (Post 1992). In this model, environmental events change the biological mechanisms that lead to mood disorders. Each time a person becomes depressed, it makes it that much easier for predispositions to express themselves on future occasions, so it takes less severe stressors to uncover them. Therefore, stressors might play a more important role in the *early* stages of mood disorders, with negative events increasing sensitivity to further episodes.

In summary, MDD is heterogeneous. The melancholic forms take severe, life-threatening forms, whereas mild to moderate depression can be thought of as "the common cold of psychiatry." If the predisposition to depression is widely distributed in the population, this helps explain why environmental changes, such as the social factors implicated in cohort effects, can cause dramatic changes in the frequency of depressive illness.

CONCLUSION

In depression, a genetic predisposition is probably a necessary but not a sufficient condition for developing overt illness. The life events preceding a depressive episode tend to be those that could be stressful for anyone, and these stressors lead to only mild or temporary impairments in most people. On the other hand, in those with a depressive diathesis, the same events lead to major psychopathology. Without stressful events, a diathesis may never become manifest. The following conclusions seem consistent with the present evidence about MDD:

1. Severe depressions (i.e., with melancholia or psychosis) do not occur without a genetic predisposition.
2. Milder cases of depression have weaker genetic predispositions, and the environment contributes more to their development.

3. Shared environmental factors, some deriving from the family environment and some from the larger social environment, may be important risk factors.
4. There is no simple causal relationship between stressful events and depression.

CHAPTER 9

ANXIETY DISORDERS AND OBSESSIVE-COMPULSIVE DISORDER

ANXIETY DISORDERS

The experience of anxiety is universal. Like depression, anxiety is a biologically programmed response to environmental stress. Its main function is to mobilize the organism to deal with danger (Nesse 2019). When there is no real danger, we can separate anxiety from fear. Some individuals have lower thresholds than others for developing anxious symptoms. We also need to understand how anxiety becomes independent of precipitating circumstances and how anxiety takes different forms: the terror of a panic attack or the constant worry of generalized anxiety disorder.

Genetic Predispositions to Anxiety Disorders

Panic disorder and generalized anxiety disorder (GAD) are the most important of the anxiety disorders seen in practice. Each has a significant heritable component. Key evidence comes from twin studies: Torgersen (1983), the first to use DSM criteria in examining twins with anxiety disorders, found that panic disorder symptoms have the highest heritability (31%). Similar findings emerged from samples of American women, one of which found a heritability of 30%–40% (Kendler et al. 1993c) and the other of 38% (Mosing et al. 2009). As for GAD, estimates of heritability generally run about 30% (Gottschalk and Domschke 2017; Kendler et al. 1992b).

However, attempts to link anxiety disorders to specific genes have not been very successful. For example, a recent genome-wide association study of anxiety disorders in veterans (Levey et al. 2020) found several significant correlations with specific alleles but did not account for most of the variance. As discussed in the previous chapter, one of the problems in studying genetic predispositions is our uncertainty about the validity of boundaries around diagnostic entities. Another is the high comorbidity between anxiety and depression. A third is whether we are measuring traits or disorders. A review by Davies et al. (2015) estimated the heritability of anxiety sensitivity, measured as a trait, at 42%.

Panic disorder and GAD have striking phenomenological differences. Panic disorder occurs in discrete episodes, whereas GAD is continuous. Patients with panic are also characterized by anticipatory anxiety and a complication of agoraphobia. Yet behavioral genetic research does not support a sharp boundary between these conditions (Kendler et al. 1987); a large overlap in genetic predispositions has been found between the two disorders, as well as with depression. In most ways, GAD functions more like a trait than a categorical disorder. It might therefore have the same relation to acute anxiety as persistent depressive disorder has to major depression. GAD is also shown to be highly comorbid with personality disorders (Blashfield et al. 1994). Until we understand the biological underpinnings of anxiety and depression, the last word cannot be said about their relationship. It would be of great theoretical interest if it turns out that a common trait predisposition can be shaped into different, albeit overlapping, symptomatic patterns by environmental patterns (Kendler et al. 1987).

One might expect the predispositions to anxiety disorders to be apparent prior to the development of overt illness. At least in some individuals, predispositions consisting of anxious traits can be observed early in life—even during infancy. Social anxiety can be identified in young children by an unusually strong fear of strangers or of new situations. This temperamental variation has been termed "behavioral inhibition" (Kagan 1994). The presence of these traits in early childhood increases the risk for anxiety disorders in adolescence (Rosenbaum et al. 1993), but long-term follow-up of children with these characteristics into adulthood has not been carried out.

Environmental Stressors in Anxiety Disorders

As was the case in mood disorders, stressors do not have a specific relationship to anxiety disorders. Underlying traits can be activated by a variety of life events. To examine the relationship of anxiety above and beyond depression, a longitudinal study of a large community sample of adolescents over a 2-year period measured the trait of anxiety sensitivity (McLaughlin and Hatzenbuehler 2009). The results showed that life events affect sensitivity and that sensitivity affects the impact of life events.

Faravelli and Pallanti (1989) reported that recent negative life events are most common before the *first* episode of panic disorder, and lower levels of stress may be required to reactivate panic symptoms once they have already occurred (i.e., a kindling mechanism). In the Virginia Twin Study (Sheerin et al. 2018), higher scores on a measure of resilience were found to be protective against GAD symptoms following further stressful life events.

In summary, causation between life events and anxiety may be bidirectional. Attachment theory (Cassidy and Shaver 2016) predicts that individuals prone to anxiety may have had more experiences of threatened or real separation and loss early in life. However, this "intergenerational transmission" of attachment patterns might be explained by traits common to parents and children. Until we can identify the biological markers for anxious traits, it will be difficult to disentangle the effects of nature and nurture.

Retrospective studies do suggest that adults with anxiety disorders have had serious difficulties in their early family life (Parker 1983). However, retrospective patient reports may reflect the tendency of individuals with serious present difficulties to describe their past as problematical. Moreover, problems in parental behaviors are nonspecific to anxiety disorders, with very similar reports coming from patients with mood disorders, personality disorders, and many other psychiatric diagnoses. We can best interpret these data as supporting the hypothesis that genetic predispositions determine whether patients are prone to panic or GAD, and environmental stressors determine when the threshold of liability is crossed.

OBSESSIVE-COMPULSIVE DISORDER

OCD has an interesting history. The radical changes in how clinicians have viewed this condition over time resemble the story of schizophrenia. Fifty years ago, obsessions and compulsions were thought of as defenses against conflicts. Today we know that OCD affects brain structure and functional connectivity (Moreira et al. 2017). We also know that the disorder is associated with strong genetic predisposition (International Obsessive Compulsive Disorder Foundation Genetics Collaborative [IOCDF-GC] and OCD Collaborative Genetics Association Studies [OCGAS] 2018).

Twin studies, including a large community study in Sweden, suggest that the symptoms of OCD have a 40%–50% heritability (Vidal-Ribas et al. 2015). As shown by genome-wide association studies, no specific genes are associated with the disorder (Mattheisen et al. 2015). Another line of evidence is that OCD has an early onset, usually in childhood and adolescence (Geller 2006). Finally, OCD has a stable cross-cultural prevalence (Staley and Wand 1995), further supporting the assumption that it has a large biological component.

Studies of environmental stressors in OCD show that adverse life events can trigger the onset of symptoms (Vidal-Ribas et al. 2015). The stressors that are most related are abuse, neglect, and family disruption, but none of these stressors explains more than 3% of the variance in outcome. In another twin study (Taylor 2011), nonshared environmental factors were also identified. In summary, OCD appears to be largely biological, with only weak evidence for psychosocial risk.

CHAPTER 10

POSTTRAUMATIC STRESS DISORDER

THE CONSTRUCT OF PTSD

Life can be marked by traumatic events, but only a minority of individuals ever develops PTSD. The perception that this disorder has become ubiquitous reflects belief systems in modern society that focus on the impact of adversity and trauma (Horwitz 2018). However, the fact that most people never experience these symptoms demonstrates the importance of gene-environment interactions.

The diagnosis of PTSD was introduced into the DSM system in 1980, following the Vietnam War (American Psychiatric Association 1980). Since then, the concept has broadened to include the effects of other traumas, such as rape or exposure to violent assaults. Yet the fact that traumatic experiences can have lasting effects has been known throughout human history. Descriptions can even be found in such classical sources as Homer's *Odyssey*. The description of a specific medical syndrome associated with trauma appeared only in the nineteenth century, however, largely as a result of observations on the effects of combat during the American Civil War (Trimble 1985). Since then, posttraumatic symptoms were described by clinicians after each of the conflicts that marked the twentieth century. In the First World War, the effects of combat exposure were called "shell shock"; in the Second World War, a similar syndrome was called "combat fatigue." The experiences of psychiatrists working with Vietnam veterans led to the present construct of PTSD

(Wolf and Mosnaim 1990). The past few decades have seen a strong revival of interest in all sorts of trauma as causes of psychopathology.

PTSD is primarily defined by recurrent intrusive recollections and a sensitivity to environmental events that resemble the original event. In DSM-5 (American Psychiatric Association 2013), posttraumatic reactions are subclassified by their time course: symptoms lasting less than a month are considered an acute stress reacrtion (i.e., *acute stress disorder*), symptoms lasting up to 3 months are termed *acute PTSD*, and symptoms lasting more than 3 months are termed *chronic PTSD*.

A large amount of research about PTSD has appeared (Bryant 2019). However, much of it suffers from two serious problems. The first is that in most studies, exposure to trauma has been measured retrospectively and not prospectively. This is a critical problem for all trauma research. Retrospective perceptions of life experience are usually influenced by present levels of symptomatology. Thus, when we ask veterans who are presently symptomatic about their war experiences, they are more likely to describe them as traumatic. When Southwick et al. (1997) followed Gulf War veterans prospectively, those who continued to have symptoms tended to remember their war experiences as more traumatic over time.

A second problem is the high comorbidity of PTSD. As Young (1995) observed, most war veteran psychiatric patients have presentations that meet criteria for many other psychiatric disorders, particularly depression and substance abuse. In addition, we cannot ignore the role that compensation plays in the continuation of posttraumatic symptoms. Yet in spite of all these complexities, some clinicians attribute the morbidity of these patients almost entirely to a history of trauma.

GENE-ENVIRONMENT MODEL OF PTSD

PTSD is one of the few categories in the DSM classification that has a putative etiological agent built into its definition. Yet no simple causal relationship exists between trauma and PTSD. The construct of PTSD also has several problems. First, how do we define *trauma*? This term has been overused to the point that almost any negative life event can be called "traumatic." We would be better advised to call events traumatic only when they consistently lead to negative effects. Yet even the most disastrous life events do not necessarily lead to pathological sequelae.

Second, how do we define *stress*? This rather vague term has been used to describe a wide variety of environmental challenges. Yet the stressfulness of life events strongly depends on the personality of the exposed person. Therefore, calling an event "stressful" need not imply that it derives from circumstances totally beyond the individual's control.

Pathological sequelae are not fully attributable to the nature of a traumatic event. It is not true that *all* individuals exposed to trauma develop posttraumatic symptoms. In fact, trauma, by itself, does *not* consistently produce PTSD, even when adverse events are severe. As reviewed by Yehuda (2002), what the data show is that the *short-term* effects of trauma are mediated largely by the nature of the event. In contrast, *long-term* effects are largely mediated by factors specific to the individual. Thus, applying DSM-5 criteria, the category with the highest prevalence among exposed populations is acute stress disorder. Acute PTSD is less common, and chronic PTSD even less so.

Combat exposure is a good example of these basic principles. In the short run, participating in combat usually produces some psychological symptoms. However, most war veterans, even those who have been in life-threatening battles, never develop PTSD. In fact, of those exposed to combat, no more than 25% develop the full clinical picture described in DSM (Laufer et al. 1984).

What determines who develops PTSD and who does not? To some extent, the *severity* of trauma is a factor. However, Lee et al. (1995), in a 50-year follow-up of Second World War veterans, found that although severity of combat exposure predicted acute PTSD, long-term symptoms were strongly related to premorbid psychopathology.

Personality traits affect the *frequency* of negative life events, determining both exposure to stressors and susceptibility to stressors. Thus, factors intrinsic to the individual could be among the most important determinants of whether trauma leads to PTSD. A second factor determining the vulnerability to trauma concerns overall predisposition to psychopathology. In a large community sample, Breslau et al. (1991) found that traumatic events are more likely to occur to individuals with personality traits of high neuroticism and high extraversion and with a previous psychiatric history.

Behavioral genetic research has provided support for the hypothesis that genetic predispositions influence whether combat veterans develop PTSD. In a large sample of twins who served in the Vietnam War, True et al. (1993) reported differences in concordance between monozygotic and dizygotic twins for each of the specific symptoms of PTSD. If *all* of the symptoms of PTSD are heritable, it cannot be a simple consequence of exposure to stress. In the same sample, Lyons et al. (1993) found that even the degree of combat exposure itself showed heritability, most probably because of the genetic component in risk taking. This is why some soldiers can turn out to be casualties or heroes.

Unlike war, the occurrence of PTSD following disasters has allowed researchers to apply prospective methodologies, in which the severity of exposure to the traumatic event can be measured at baseline instead of being assessed retrospectively years later. In a classical study of Australian firefighters, McFarlane (1990) found that over time, the longer symptoms remained, the less they were accounted for by exposure to trauma and the more they were accounted for by predispositions. As in other research, vulnerability to PTSD depended on personality traits of neuroticism or conflict avoidance, as well as on either a family history or a history of psychiatric illness.

Later behavioral genetic studies (e.g., Stein et al. 2002) have replicated these findings. In a large-scale genome-wide association study, Duncan et al. (2018) found a large heritable component (25% overall and at least 50% in women), which was shared with several other major psychiatric disorders. In summary, the symptoms of PTSD result from the triggering of responses to which the individual is already predisposed or an exacerbation of symptoms that had previously been present. Research indicates that although *acute* PTSD can often be accounted for by exposure to trauma, *chronic* PTSD cannot. Chronicity derives from predisposing factors, and resilience factors can protect exposed individuals against chronicity.

CHILDHOOD TRAUMA

When trauma occurs at a defined moment in time, the course of post-traumatic symptoms can be followed prospectively. If, on the other hand, traumatic events have occurred at some point in the past, we are presented with serious methodological problems. Given the effects of all possible intervening events, it becomes very difficult to attribute psychopathology to temporally distant stressors. This problem raises serious doubts about the claims, based entirely on retrospective studies, that childhood trauma consistently causes PTSD or that traumatic events in childhood lead to predictable long-term sequelae.

A large number of studies using retrospective designs have claimed to document associations between childhood trauma and adult psychopathology. For example, high rates of trauma of childhood sexual abuse and physical abuse have been reported with great frequency by some groups of patients. One could interpret these reports as showing that childhood trauma is indeed an important risk factor. However, it is equally possible that these associations are due to other risks that have not been examined.

Community surveys of the long-term sequelae of childhood trauma put these issues in perspective. It has been known for decades that the great majority of survivors of childhood sexual abuse have no measurable psychopathology (Browne and Finkelhor 1986; Fergusson et al. 1996) and that the same is true for physical abuse (Malinosky-Rummell and Hansen 1993). Thus, there are many more nonpatients than patients with trauma histories. This not to say that these experiences have no effect. Fergusson et al. (1996b) concluded that "the weight of the evidence points to the conclusion that CSA [child sexual abuse] may play a significant, but not overwhelmingly strong, role in determining individual vulnerability to psychiatric disorder" (p. 1373).

As in adult PTSD, exposure to trauma is a necessary but not a sufficient condition for the development of symptoms. Associations between child abuse histories and adult disorders are correlational and not necessarily causal. Moreover, trauma is not one thing but many things. The sequelae of abuse depend very much on severity of exposure and what exactly happened. Therefore, to understand the impact of any adverse experience, we must consider its *parameters.*

As discussed in Chapter 3, risk depends on severity of exposure, which is an important predictor of the long-term effects of all adversities during childhood (Rutter 1987a). In childhood sexual abuse, the most powerful predictor of sequelae includes the perpetrator being a member of the same family (especially father–daughter incest), abuse that is more frequent and goes on for longer, and the nature of the sexual contact (Browne and Finkelhor 1986). However, even when these severity parameters are taken into account, the majority of children exposed to sexual abuse do not develop significant psychopathology.

Clinicians should also keep in mind that single traumatic experiences in childhood do not usually lead to mental disorders, whereas multiple negative events tend to lead to cumulative effects that significantly increase the risk for psychopathology (Rutter 1987a). Any one adverse event in childhood interacts with many other life experiences. Associations between single events and sequelae can give us the mistaken impression that single incidents have enormous consequences. Even multiple adversities have a statistical relationship to outcome and do not always produce sequelae.

This is why the ICD-11 (World Health Organization 2019) made a mistake in adding a new diagnosis of complex PTSD based on the concept of "complex trauma." The idea is that when adversities are multiple and long-lasting, they produce a unique syndrome that resembles the clinical picture of borderline personality disorder. However, as I discuss later in Chapter 13, that disorder has a large heritable component.

The complex trauma construct supports the mistaken impression that symptoms similar to borderline personality disorder are mainly due to trauma and that cumulative traumatic events usually lead to this clinical syndrome.

All empirical findings about the impact of trauma point to the importance of resilience (Rutter 2012). To the extent that other experiences are positive, the child will be more likely to be resilient, but there are also genetic factors in resilience. Some relate to neurobiological systems (Feder et al. 2009). Personality traits in children may determine environmental sensitivity—that is, whether they are "orchids" or "dandelions" (Boyce 2019).

Other mechanisms of intergenerational transmission of trauma could involve epigenetics (Sheerin et al. 2017; Yehuda and Lehrner 2018). Yehuda et al. (2014) also showed that PTSD in parents can influence epigenetic regulation of the glucocorticoid receptor gene in the children of Holocaust survivors. The mechanism involves regulation of glucocorticoids, and one of the reasons epigenetic effects can be found in the third generation is because the gametes of future grandchildren are already present in their parents.

Yet although PTSD research has continued to progress, we need to be careful about what we label "traumatic" events that have consequences. Measurements of trauma are based on retrospective reports, yet the way we remember things, as well as the way we explain our memories, is very much a function of our personality as well as how we are functioning later on in life. It is not surprising, therefore, that when behavioral geneticists examine standard self-report instruments about childhood experience in twins, many of which purport to be measures of the environment, a substantial heritable component affects scores on all these scales (Plomin 1994).

Some aspects of rearing may be more affected by the child's personality than others. Thus, in studies of twins reporting on how their parents raised them (Rowe 1981), a large heritable component affected how adults remembered parental affection (but not control). The most likely explanation is that positive temperamental characteristics in *children* elicit more affection from parents, whereas the way parents control their children depends on personality traits of the *parents*.

Clinicians need to understand the problems with the accuracy of recollections before coming to firm conclusions about historical material presented in psychotherapy. The development of false memories in psychotherapy has been a serious problem. It is unlikely that patients *want* to make up stories about being abused as children. Recollections of experiences are shaped by suggestions coming from many sources, including books, media, and previous therapists (Loftus 1993). Memories are not accurate recordings of the past but largely consist of reconstructed narratives.

In spite of all these problems, PTSD deserves its place in the psychiatric nomenclature. In accord with prominent psychosocial risk factors in its etiology, and taking into account the fact that resilience is a factor and that genes do not fully determine symptoms, PTSD has been found to be treatable with evidence-based psychotherapies (Watkins et al. 2018).

CONCLUSION

PTSD, which seems at first glance to fit a primarily environmental model of psychopathology, turns out instead to demonstrate the necessity for a gene-environment model. However dramatic the symptoms, and however deserving these patients are of our concern, we need to address the role of predispositions and prior psychopathology. These factors are crucial for understanding why traumatic events do not always have long-term effects. The same principle applies to adult patients who report childhood trauma. Traumatic stressors do not usually produce lasting psychopathology on their own but act to unleash preexisting vulnerabilities.

CHAPTER 11

― EATING DISORDERS

THE TWO main categories of eating disorder, anorexia nervosa and bulimia nervosa, are different. Patients with anorexia restrict eating, whereas those with bulimia lose control of intake. These disorders also overlap in some cases; for example, patients with both anorexia and binges are more like bulimia than like typical anorexia.

Many people worry about their weight, but few ever develop eating disorders. Other risk factors determine whether attitudes about body image are normal or pathological. Both anorexia and bulimia nervosa are highly influenced by social risk factors. The first clinical description of anorexia nervosa (Gull 1873) was published in the nineteenth century, and typical cases can be identified from the medical literature. The disorder has been on the increase; epidemiological studies (Smink et al. 2012) find that prevalence is about 0.6%, with the most striking increases occurring in adolescent girls and young adults.

ANOREXIA NERVOSA

Genetic Predispositions

Anorexia nervosa can be a life-threatening disease. As with other mental disorders, we would expect that the more severe an illness is, and the earlier in life it appears, the more likely it is to have a strong genetic predisposition. Evidence supports this expectation: one review found the heritability of anorexia to lie between 40% and 60% (Trace et al. 2013), but earlier twin studies had found a heritability as high as 88% (Bulik et al. 2000). The reason for this discrepancy probably lies in variation between samples. Two genome-wide association studies (Baker et al. 2017; Li et al. 2017) identified a few significant loci, but the genetic risk was shared with several other mental disorders. Another recent study found that genetic factors may contribute to risk because of their effects of metabolism (Hübel et al. 2019).

Obesity is not frequent among the relatives of patients with anorexia (Treasure and Holland 1995). This goes along with the fact that instead of being prone to weight gain, patients with anorexia are "restrictors" in their eating behavior, and these traits are associated with comorbidity for personality disorders in the anxious cluster associated with compulsive personality traits and perfectionism. (Treasure and Holland 1995). This conclusion has been supported by a meta-analysis (Dahlenburg et al. 2019), which also suggested that perfectionism is a risk for eating disorders of all kind.

Psychosocial Risk Factors

Families may play a role in the risk for anorexia, but one review found risk factors not specific to the disorder (i.e., maternal concern about child weight, children's level of family satisfaction, family exposure to stress) (Allen et al. 2014). Råstam and Gillberg (1991) failed to find any "typical" family structure associated with anorexia. It may be useful to see this disorder as a culture-bound syndrome (Prince and Tcheng-Laroche 1987); diagnoses that exist only in specific cultural settings can be thought of, at least from our own perspective, as "exotic." However, our Western culture also leads to the molding of universal vulnerabilities.

The best explanation of the increased prevalence of eating disorders in modern societies is that they derive from a culturally shaped pursuit of thinness (Garner and Garfinkel 1985). Thinness is rarely a goal in cultures that have known starvation or high levels of mortality in children, where children are seen as healthier when they are slightly overweight. Social forces, by encouraging women to seek unrealistic levels of slimness, lower the threshold for excessive concerns about body image. In an apocryphal story, Duchess of Windsor Wallis Simpson is said to have remarked, "A woman can never be too rich or too thin."

These trends are particularly strong in North American and European societies. One only has to browse through any bookstore to appreciate how important dieting has become in our culture. These pressures are also more common in the upper classes. The pervasive pursuit of thinness among women in developed countries can be understood as a form of *sexual selection*, in which a trait can be contrary to survival but is favored in the short run if it increases the likelihood of finding a mate. Like the tail of the peacock, exaggerated thinness is a "super-normal stimulus" (Cronin 1991).

Eating disorders are rarely seen in traditional societies, but this situation is changing as cultures around the globe undergo modernization. Eating disorders have been diagnosed for the first time in the children of immigrants to developed countries (DiNicola 1990). In developed societies in which hunger is relatively unknown, children rarely die, so milder degrees of obesity can be seen by young females as reducing their sexual attractiveness. For this reason, the overwhelmingly higher prevalence of eating disorders in women should not be surprising.

In the past, the structure of European societies resembled in most ways that of today's developing countries, and concerns with body image were much less common. As documented by historians (Brumberg 1988), cases of self-starvation prior to the nineteenth century were usually related to excessive religious preoccupation. Today. we have different sociocultural challenges associated with modernity to which patients with anorexia nervosa are more susceptible.

BULIMIA NERVOSA

Genetic Predispositions

Bulimia nervosa is a less dangerous illness than anorexia. Its boundaries with abnormal eating behavior are fuzzy, and it is much more prevalent than anorexia. We might therefore expect it to be less heritable. Research findings tend to confirm these expectations. The Virginia Twin Study reported a heritability of 50%–55% (Kendler et al. 1991), but a later study from the same sample (Bulik et al. 2000) reported only 28%. Genome-wide association studies have been largely negative (Mayhew et al. 2018). The overall conclusion at this point is that genetic factors in bulimia nervosa are weaker than in anorexia.

These contradictions reflect the heterogeneity of bulimia. This illness, once quite rare, has become common, with a prevalence of 1%–4% (Mayhew et al. 2018). An association has been found between bulimia and a vulnerability to becoming overweight, and obesity is unusually common among the relatives of these patients (Treasure and Holland 1995). Patients are trying to maintain their weight below a natural "set point." Some people always have trouble maintaining their weight, whereas others remain svelte without difficulty. In an adoption study, Stunkard et al. (1986) found the tendency to obesity to be heritable.

In a Darwinian context, this finding should not be surprising. A trait favoring fat storage would have been very useful in the environment of evolutionary adaptiveness. Although those who stayed thin would be generally healthier under normal conditions, those with a genetic tendency to obesity would have a greater capacity to store calories. This would therefore better protect them against inevitable food shortages (Nesse and Williams 1994). These genetic variations would not have caused obesity in environments in which there was little excess food to be eaten and in which regular exercise was not simply an elective health-promoting activity but a necessity for survival. In modern societies, in which food is abundant and exercise can be avoided, there are bound to be more obese individuals. The social pressure to be thin, particularly among women, is what leads many to make serious efforts to lose weight. Excessive dieting, leading to hunger, can be a triggering factor in bulimia nervosa.

The second element in the predisposition to bulimia nervosa involves personality traits. Personality structures among patients with bulimia are variable, although many have traits of emotional dysregulation and impulsivity related to borderline personality disorder (Peterson et al. 2010; Rosenvinge et al. 2000). In bulimia, symptoms are the opposite of the restriction seen in anorexia, with a loss of control and an inability to stop a binge once it starts. It therefore resembles substance use disorders. Bulimia therefore contrasts with the compulsive traits commonly seen in anorexia.

Psychosocial Risk Factors

No clear boundary has been defined between bulimia nervosa and abnormal eating behavior, and the twin study by Kendler et al. (1991a) found that the risk factors for narrowly defined bulimia and binge eating are very similar. Their data fit a multiple-threshold model, with one threshold for a more severe form of disorder and another for a less severe form. Steiger et al. (2007) documented risk factors of child maltreatment as well as growing up in families that are high in conflict, low in cohesion, and low in emotional responsiveness. This picture is rather similar to what has been described in borderline personality disorder (see Chapter 13).

GENE-ENVIRONMENT INTERACTIONS IN EATING DISORDERS

In summary, both anorexia nervosa and bulimia nervosa are complex disorders that develop in the presence of a combination of biological predispositions, psychological stressors, and powerful social influences. Patients with anorexia show a stronger genetic predisposition toward restriction of eating to obtain control. These features generally become apparent in adolescence, with all its developmental changes. Patients with bulimia show emotion dysregulation and impulsive traits. This leads them to bypass a natural set point that would make them slightly overweight. The problem in both disorders is amplified by a response to the cultural pursuit of thinness.

CHAPTER 12

SUBSTANCE-RELATED AND ADDICTIVE DISORDERS

Sᴜʙꜱᴛᴀɴᴄᴇ ᴀʙᴜꜱᴇ is one of the most common of all mental disorders, although only some of these patients present to psychiatrists. This chapter focuses mostly on alcoholism, which has attracted the most research and has a 12-month prevalence of 14% in males (Grant et al. 2015; Robins and Regier 1991).

GENETIC PREDISPOSITIONS TO SUBSTANCE USE

A genetic predisposition to alcoholism has long been understood, and research in this area is substantial (Schuckit 2014). However, no clear cutoff point has been found between increased consumption of alcohol, problem drinking, and clinically diagnosable alcoholism. Many decades ago, Jellinek (1960) hypothesized different forms of alcoholism, some having a later onset and being less familial and others having an earlier onset and being more familial. A contemporary version of this classification emerged from adoption studies of alcoholism conducted in Scandinavia (Sigvardsson et al. 1996). The findings also pointed to two independently heritable types of alcohol abuse. "Type 1 alcoholism" has a later onset, affects both sexes, and is determined by both genetic and environmental factors. "Type 2 alcoholism" has an early onset, affects only men, is associated with criminality, and is more strongly determined by genetic factors.

Large-scale population-based twin studies (Kendler and Prescott 2006) have demonstrated that problem drinking has a large genetic effect, accounting for about 50% of the variance in average weekly consumption of alcohol. Additional evidence for a biological predisposition to alcoholism comes from the series of adoption studies conducted in Scandinavia, as well as from replications in North American samples (Goodwin and Warnock 1991). Adoptees who have a biological parent with alcoholism are much more likely to develop alcoholism themselves. Those with a liability to alcoholism are also more likely to experience drinking alcohol as pleasurable, even on the first exposure (Schuckit 1986) and more likely to become dependent on the substance over time. This is a good example of how genes influence both susceptibility to the environment and exposure to environmental risk factors. The other side of this coin is that those who have an unpleasant reaction to alcohol are less likely to become addicted. One dysphoric reaction is the "oriental flush," an autonomic reaction more common in East Asian populations (Goodwin and Warnock 1991), which might partially explain a lower prevalence of alcoholism.

Alcoholism is also another case in which an early onset of illness is a marker for a stronger genetic predisposition. Buydens-Branchey et al. (1989) found that an onset of alcohol abuse before age 20 years in men is associated with higher rates of paternal alcoholism. The pattern of father–son transmission in alcoholism has been an important focus of research. Having a father with alcoholism also limits the lifespan (Landberg et al. 2018). The sons of men with alcoholism, but not necessarily daughters, show several differences from control subjects: they have a much greater tolerance for alcohol, have differences in their event-related potentials as measured by electroencephalography, and also demonstrate abnormalities on neuropsychological testing (Schuckit 1986).

Tarter et al. (1995) studied the temperamental factors that place individuals at risk for alcoholism, including increased behavioral activity, a short attention span, a decreased ability to be soothed, increased harm avoidance, increased novelty seeking, and increased sociability. These traits, it should be noted, are also relevant for many other disorders, such as ADHD and antisocial personality disorder, any of which can be comorbid with alcoholism. The precursors of addiction need not involve substance use, but can instead involve a range of externalizing and internalizing disorders. As shown by a meta-analysis, a number of childhood psychiatric disorders, including ADHD, conduct disorder, oppositional defiant disorder, and depression, are associated with an outcome of at least one substance-related disorder (Groenman et al. 2017).

In summary, a vulnerability to alcoholism is strongly heritable. However, we do not know *what* is inherited. Individual differences in the effects of alcohol on the brain could be the effects of a specific predisposition or could depend on the presence of one or several personality traits. We also do not know whether these predispositions are specific to alcohol or are equally associated with an increased risk for abusing other substances.

Alcoholism has a striking differential in sex prevalence. One of the hypotheses has been that individuals with alcoholism are really "treating" themselves for depression. Alcoholism and depression can run in the same families, suggesting that they might be different expressions of the same predisposition. One piece of evidence supporting this view is that among the Amish of Pennsylvania, a group in which alcoholism is rare and the female preponderance for severe depression seen in most American populations is not found (Egeland and Hostetter 1983).

We do not know precisely how genes raise the risk for alcoholism. Wang et al. (2012) suggested that the "most well-established genetic factors associated with alcohol dependence are in the genes encoding alcohol dehydrogenase (ADH), which oxidizes alcohol to acetaldehyde, and aldehyde dehydrogenase (ALDH2), which oxidizes acetaldehyde to acetate" (p. 258), However, these polymorphisms are relatively uncommon. Genome-wide association studies on alcoholism have been inconclusive (Clarke et al. 2017). Similarly, genome-wide association studies of stimulant and opioid use disorders report only suggestive findings that require replication (Jensen 2016).

Bierut (2011) noted that genetic studies have been less successful in predicting use but better at identifying factors that influence the transition to dependence. The choice of substance does not seem to be related to heritable risk. Kendler et al. (2003), using data from the Virginia Twin Study, concluded that both the genetic and shared environmental effects on risk for the use and misuse of six classes of illicit substances were nonspecific in their effect. Finally, it should be kept in mind that the genes that increase risk for substance use disorders also have powerful effects on psychosocial functioning. For example, Kendler et al. (2017) found that genetic differences can predict divorce, largely because of their effects on alcohol use disorder.

ENVIRONMENTAL RISK FACTORS FOR SUBSTANCE ABUSE

Many assume that alcoholism must have roots in an unhappy childhood. Retrospective studies in which patients are asked about their life experiences are likely to elicit such recollections. However, this method fails to separate the effects of genetics and environment. Moreover, patients with alcoholism are known for their tendency to blame others, not excluding their parents, for their current problems. We need to conduct prospective research in which childhood variables are measured prior to the onset of substance abuse.

We still do not have many studies in which young children have been followed into adulthood to see whether they develop alcoholism. Some years ago, Vaillant (1995) followed a group of adolescents who had not yet developed alcoholism, assessing their family background retrospectively and following the cohort prospectively for many years. Family history was a good predictor of later alcoholism, but the data failed to show that the quality of childhood experience was related to addiction in adulthood. Although some who eventually developed alcoholism had had behavioral problems in childhood and adolescence, most were asymptomatic prior to developing addiction. Moreover, when those with alcoholism stopped drinking, they did not necessarily have residual symptoms (Vaillant 1995). If, on the other hand, they returned to alcohol, their previous degree of behavioral psychopathology returned in all its severity. These findings suggest that in those who are susceptible to substance abuse, psychopathology can be the *result* of the addiction rather than its cause.

One of the largest studies designed to predict substance use and antisocial behavior was conducted by Richard Tremblay at the University of Montreal. The results, drawn from several prospectively followed cohorts, supported the conclusion that predispositions are a necessary cause of alcoholism but also leave room for environmental factors. Carbonneau et al. (2018) reported that paternal alcoholism is a risk regardless of whether the father lives with the family. Dobkin et al. (1997) found that early use of alcohol predicts later problems and that mothers' lack of nurturance was also a factor. Generalizing the findings to other substances, Rioux et al. (2018a) reported that an early age of cannabis use, reinforced by pathological peer groups, is associated with abuse of this drug in adolescence.

Because substance use can affect both humans and other species, it is therefore one of the few mental disorders for which researchers can develop animal models (Spanagel 2017). The pharmacological effects of substances largely depend on their ability to tap into existing neurochemical mechanisms. Yet why do people prefer one substance over another? After all, some are stimulating and others are sedating, but many patients we see have polysubstance abuse. The evidence suggests that a common predisposition for many types of substance abuse. This trait has been called an "addictive personality."

Evidence has shown that substance abuse is linked to impulsive personality traits, leading to an inability to control intake. Impulsive traits and sensation seeking could also help explain the high comorbidity between substance abuse and personality disorders (Mitchell and Potenza 2014). Those who are susceptible to substance abuse of any kind could have chronic dysphoria, leading them to use drugs as a form of self-medication. In this view, addiction would develop when hyperreactivity to stress is specifically buffered by the intake of a substance.

SOCIOCULTURAL FACTORS IN SUBSTANCE USE

Some of the most important environmental factors mediating the expression of a predisposition to alcohol are social. We see substance use in some form in every society. Yet different cultures can either promote or suppress substance abuse, and the choice of a substance may also be determined by sociocultural factors. A good deal of evidence supports this hypothesis (Oetting et al. 1998). Very wide cross-national differences, as well as cohort effects, have been found that affect the choice of substances and the extent to which they will be abused.

Alcohol has always been, and continues to be, the substance of choice in most cultures throughout human history. However, in the past, opioid dependence was highly endemic in China, and it has returned as a major cause of addiction in North America. After a long period of declining use, cocaine also became a serious clinical problem in many Western countries. Cultural norms encourage substance use by associating its use with reinforcing interpersonal relationships. The primary example consists of the male bonding rituals associated with drinking in many societies. Cultures can also discourage substance use, either by enforcing sanctions and prohibitions against abuse or by associating its use with activities in which the role of the substance is secondary, such as taking alcohol only with meals.

Although no society has been described in which alcoholism is totally absent, striking differences can be found in its prevalence in countries around the world (Helzer and Canino 1992). Some of the cross-cultural differences in alcoholism might be accounted for by racial differences associated with genetically determined dysphoric physical effects whenever alcohol is imbibed (Goodwin and Warnock 1991). However, such explanations cannot account for other cross-national differences, such as the high rate of alcoholism in France and much lower rate in Italy. Most likely, social factors are responsible for these differences.

Genetic predispositions to alcoholism can be either suppressed or amplified by social attitudes toward drinking. These social factors include where people drink (e.g., in bars or at the dinner table) as well as whether heavy drinking is encouraged. We cannot explain the preponderance of males with alcoholism entirely on the basis of predispositions, and social factors in males probably shape their vulnerability to overt alcoholism. In many societies, men drink heavily to establish bonding, whereas women do not. Many men are willing to pay that price.

In summary, a combination of genetic predisposition, exposure to the substance, and social reinforcements accounts for the development of alcoholism in men. Women, in whom alcohol use is much more likely to be used as self-medication, probably have a different pathway to alcohol abuse. Similar principles probably apply to other forms of substance abuse, which is associated with unstable families and poverty (Kendler and Prescott 2006).

GENES AND ENVIRONMENT IN SUBSTANCE ABUSE

Substance abuse provides one of the best-documented examples of the gene-environment model in psychopathology. Research evidence shows that there are genetic predispositions to alcoholism and that social factors strongly influence the prevalence of abuse. Future investigations will probably support a similar model for other forms of substance abuse. In summary, the most parsimonious explanation of the data on alcoholism is:

1. Those with the strongest predisposition may develop the disorder in any cultural setting where the substance is available.
2. When the culture encourages excessive drinking, those with weaker predispositions will also be affected, and alcoholism will be more common.
3. The most important risk factor for alcoholism is a strong family history, especially in fathers.

CHAPTER 13

PERSONALITY DISORDERS

PROBLEMS OF DIAGNOSIS AND CLASSIFICATION

Personality disorder describes a long-term pattern of dysfunction in emotions, thoughts, and relationships that is not attributable to other mental disorders. It is often a pathological exaggeration of normal personality traits. Thus, patients rarely come for a personality disorder itself but instead seek treatment for accompanying symptoms such as depression or anxiety. Clinicians who are trained to focus on symptoms may have difficulty making these diagnoses. Nonetheless, personality disorders are among the most common problems seen in clinics and emergency departments. Community studies suggest that their prevalence in the general population is about 10% (Lenzenweger 2008). Clinical prevalence of any personality disorder can be as high as 50% (Zimmerman et al. 2008). Borderline personality disorder (BPD) is the most clinically important category and has been the subject of the most research, with thousands of published papers. For this reason, this chapter focuses on that category.

BPD differs from most other personality disorders in having prominent symptoms such as depression, anxiety, mood instability, self-harm, substance use, and suicidality. BPD is also characterized by highly problematic intimate relationships. Even so, Zimmerman and Mattia (1999) found that many cases are missed and that clinicians tend to see these patients as having bipolar or unipolar mood disorders.

Antisocial personality disorder is most familiar to forensic psychiatrists, and about one-third of prisoners meet criteria (Black et al. 2010). These cases begin with conduct disorder, which child psychiatrists often see, but adults with antisocial personality disorder do not necessarily present to clinics. The other categories of personality disorder listed in DSM-5 (Section II) are much less researched (American Psychiatric Association 2013). A strong movement has grown among personality disorder researchers to replace many if not all of them. The theoretical basis of that change is that if personality traits and personality disorders lie on a continuum, clinical cases can be based on the scoring of dimensions of personality.

As a result, there are multiple methods of diagnosing personality disorders. In DSM-5, Section II repeats the classification developed for previous editions of the manual, but Section III presents the alternative model of personality disorders, in which categorical diagnoses are built on quantitative measures of clinically observed traits (Hopwood et al. 2019). In this "hybrid" model, the number of categories has been reduced from 10 to 6. Since its introduction in 2013, the alternative model has the subject of much research (Zimmermann et al. 2019) and could eventually become the official system of classification. ICD-11 has taken the more radical step of eliminating categories entirely in favor of a trait system with five dimensions as well as measures of severity (Tyrer et al. 2011; World Health Organization 2019). However, after pushback from BPD researchers in Europe and America, the final version allows identification of a "borderline pattern," which closely resembles the DSM definition of that disorder.

PERSONALITY TRAITS

Development of a personality disorder involves a progression from traits to disorders. These pathways depend on the strength of genetic predispositions, the intensity of environmental stressors, and their interactions. Studies of the effects of genes and environment on traits and disorders in the same population do not support a simple model of continuity (Kendler et al. 2019). Nonetheless, individual differences in traits, which reflect inborn temperament, can determine the form that personality disorders take. In the past, psychological theories assumed that abnormal personality is *largely* environmental in origin and that the stability of personality over time could be explained by roots in early childhood experience. At the other extreme, biological theories proposed that personality disorders are a reflection of inborn chemical imbalances (Cloninger 1987). Both views are mistaken. Personality disorder is a prime example of interactions between nature and nurture.

Each individual has a unique way of responding to environmental challenges. These characteristics constitute what is commonly called "personality." We can define personality *traits* as patterns of behavior, emotion, and cognition that remain consistent from one situation to another (Rutter 1987b). Traits show a great deal of variability between individuals. These characteristics can be identified early in life and tend to remain relatively stable over a lifetime (Widiger and Costa 2013).

Several schemas have been developed to describe personality traits (also called *dimensions*, reflecting how they are measured). Most of these systems are based on data drawn from self-report measures in community and clinical populations. By means of factor analysis, questionnaire items are grouped into scorable dimensional scales. Some classifications describe *broad* dimensions derived from the study of variability in normal personality. The most widely used schema is the Five-Factor Model (Widiger and Costa 2013), which defines traits of *extraversion, neuroticism, agreeableness, openness to experience,* and *conscientiousness,* sometimes called the "big five." These dimensions usefully describe normal personality and can also account for some of the symptoms seen in patients with personality disorders. There are also five factors (although not quite the same ones) in the diagnostic systems for personality disorders in DSM-5, Section III, and in ICD-11 (World Health Organization 2019).

Personality traits, however defined, are heritable, with nearly 50% of variance between individuals depending on genetic influences (Plomin et al. 2013). Adoption studies show that monozygotic twins raised apart show striking similarities in personality traits (Tellegen et al. 1988). These trait profiles underlie personality disorders. Traits are based, in turn, on inborn temperament but are further shaped during development by social learning (Rutter 1987b). With few exceptions, temperament is a limiting factor. For example, introverts can become less shy, but they do not become extraverts.

Temperament describes behavioral dispositions at birth that persist later in life. For example, infants can be more or less active, more or less socially responsive, more or less fearful, and more or less irritable. Chess and Thomas (1984) developed a model with three types—easy, difficult, and slow to warm up—but it is better to score temperament using dimensions. Rothbart et al. (2000) used a model describing three dimensions of temperament: positive emotionality, negative emotionality, and constraint.

Temperament in children is not stable until age 5, only modestly stable before adolescence (Bornstein et al. 2015), and not fully stable until age 30 (Shiner 2009). Thus, temperament is strongly genetic but can be modified by the environment. By and large, extreme temperaments are stronger predictors of pathology emerging later in development. Infants who are extremely irritable or extremely fearful are more likely to remain so, leading to problematical behaviors later in development (Kagan 1994). Children with increased fearfulness and irritability tend to have higher neuroticism as adults; children with increased activity level and positive affectivity tend to become more extraverted; children with attentional persistence tend to become more conscientious; and children who are easily prone to distress tend to have difficulties with attachment (Shiner 2009). Another line of evidence supporting biological factors in personality is that broad dimensions of personality are the same in many different cultures (Widiger and Costa 2013).

ENVIRONMENTAL FACTORS IN PERSONALITY

Genes are not the whole story; 50% of the variance in personality traits remains attributable to the environment. The question is, what kinds of environmental events can account for the high level of differences in personality between children raised in the same families and the same neighborhoods (Dunn and Plomin 1990)? The environmental factors shaping personality can be partly understood through social learning theory (Bandura 1977). This model hypothesizes that parents influence their children's personality through two mechanisms: 1) direct reinforcement of behaviors and 2) the child's imitation of observed parental behaviors. The model can also be applied to influences from a social community.

However, as most parents learn from their own experience, their influence has limits. Children are not clay to be shaped by parental care but have their own innate personalities. The traits of siblings living in the same family may resemble each other little more than if they came from different families (Dunn and Plomin 1990). This is probably why most parents with more than one child come to believe in genetics.

One of the surprising findings of twin research concerns the source of environmental influences on personality. As with most traits, they are largely "unshared"—that is, not related to living in the same family (Plomin et al. 2013). Unshared environmental effects could have a number of possible explanations: siblings receiving differential treatment from parents or taking on different niches in the family; individuals with different personality traits perceiving the same environment differently; or social and community factors outside the family shaping traits. All these mechanisms could be operative but are not readily disentangled.

Some of the residual variance in personality traits reflects interactions between genes and environment. Children influence the quality of their own environment by shaping the responses of others to conform to their own traits (Scarr and McCartney 1983). On the positive side, intelligent children seek out a stimulating environment. On the negative side, temperamental abnormalities in children are amplified by the difficulties they create for parents and peers (Rutter 1987b). Moreover, temperamentally irritable and impulsive children are more likely to have adverse experiences, both inside and outside the family (Rutter and Quinton 1984). The effects of temperament on personality are to "bend the twig," or set limits on what characteristics can eventually predominate in an individual. The discontinuities in personality over time point to interactions between parenting and temperament (i.e., "goodness of fit") (Chess and Thomas 1984).

PERSONALITY TRAITS AND PERSONALITY DISORDERS

If personality disorders are pathological exaggerations of normal traits, the relation between traits and disorders must involve a process of *amplification*. If that view is correct, there should be no sharp break between normal personality and pathological personality. Traits would only become disorders at some cutoff point at which they cause significant dysfunction. For example, low conscientiousness can be amplified into a destructive pattern of impulsivity, seen in Cluster B personality disorders in DSM-5, whereas high conscientiousness is associated with compulsive personality disorder.

This model is suitable for most but not all personality disorders. BPD is different. It is rooted in traits of emotional dysregulation (Linehan 1993) as well as impulsivity (Crowell et al. 2009), but BPD leads to behaviors not seen in normal personality (e.g., recurrent suicide attempts and self-harm). It also has a very wide comorbidity and can be seen as a highly symptomatic major mental disorder.

For other personality disorders, using dimensional measures of personality, the concept continuity between traits and disorders has been supported by empirical research (Hopwood et al. 2019). By and large, a wide range of variability in personality is compatible with normality. The world has room for extraverts and introverts, for those who worry and those who do not, for those who are emotional and those who are not, and for those who are cautious and for those more likely to act on impulse. Many patterns of behavior can be adaptive when applied in appropriate circumstances yet maladaptive when applied in inappropriate circumstances. Thus, extraverts tend to thrive in a setting that requires sociability but may have more difficulty when not receiving social reinforcement. Introverts are productive in settings that require a capacity to work alone but can be in danger of becoming overly isolated. People who worry are more likely to see trouble before it hits them, but they may also anticipate troubles that are unlikely to occur. People who do not worry can have a better life, but only as long as all goes well, because they are not prepared for adversity. People who are highly emotional can also feel more joyous and alive than others, but people who are relatively unemotional are better able to tolerate hard times. People who are cautious make fewer mistakes, whereas people who are impulsive tend to fare better in situations when a rapid response is required.

Personality traits are therefore alternative evolutionary strategies, each of which is more or less adaptive depending on environmental demands (Beck et al. 2014; Brune 2015; Nesse 2019). It is when these traits are discordant with social expectations that psychopathology ensues. Traits that do not meet social demands will significantly interfere with functioning. Moreover, when traits are used rigidly and maladaptively, they lead to even more dysfunction.

Eventually, when traits are amplified to the point of dysfunction, the clinical picture can come to meet the criteria for the general definition of a personality disorder. These criteria describe enduring patterns of inner experience and behavior that deviate from cultural expectations, that are inflexible and pervasive, that lead to clinically significant distress or impairment, and that are stable over time. In understanding this process, it is important to keep in mind that no single etiological factor is a sufficient cause of personality disorders. Biological, psychological, and social factors are all involved, and the process depends on multiple risk factors. These risks can also be buffered by protective factors, making the amplification of traits less likely. The type of personality disorder that develops depends on trait profiles.

GENETIC PREDISPOSITIONS FOR PERSONALITY DISORDERS

Predisposing genetic factors in personality disorders are demonstrated by behavioral genetic data (Distel et al. 2008; Reichborn-Kjennerud et al. 2013; Torgersen et al. 2012). Nearly half of the variance affecting personality disorder is heritable. However, attempts to establish links with specific genes have found only weak relationships and have generally not been replicated (Paris 2020). The largest body of behavior genetic research has focused on BPD. Moreover, the trait most associated with BPD, affective instability (or emotion dysregulation), has a similar heritability of 40%–50% (Jang et al. 1996).

The findings are supported by family history research. Although we do not often see family members with the same diagnosis, first-degree relatives tend to have subsyndromal pathology, particularly substance abuse and antisocial personality (White et al. 2003). In a sample of twins followed longitudinally, Bornovalova et al. (2009) found genetic factors were stronger predictors of BPD features across the course of adolescence than earlier in development. These are the years when BPD becomes clinically apparent.

A genome-wide association study of BPD identified hundreds of interacting genes related to the disorder, as well as genetic overlap with bipolar disorder, major depression, and schizophrenia (Witt et al. 2017). Evidently, genetic risk is not specific to BPD but is shared with other mental disorders. Although former optimism that future advances in technology could identify biological markers for personality disorders, we have found almost nothing, as is the case for almost all DSM-5 disorders.

By and large, personality disorders develop in people with predisposing traits. In one of our own studies (Laporte et al. 2011), we examined sisters of patients with BPD who grew up in the same dysfunctional families to see if they also developed BPD. In more than 90% of cases, they did not; instead, trait profiles were the best predictor of a personality disorder. In summary, genetically based temperamental factors are necessary but not sufficient causes of personality disorders.

PSYCHOLOGICAL RISK FACTORS IN PERSONALITY DISORDERS

Patients with personality disorders report an unusually large number of negative childhood experiences. They describe adversities such as early separation or loss, abnormalities in parenting, emotional neglect, and traumatic experiences such as child abuse. Not all patients report these problems, but among those who do, the common factor may be family dysfunction (Paris 2020). It should be kept in mind that most of the findings from research on the psychological factors of personality disorders depend on the validity of retrospective reports of childhood experiences. In view of the vagaries of long-term memory and the tendency for perceptions of the past to be filtered through the present, we must view the evidence with caution. Moreover, the tendency to blame parents for life problems can be reinforced by psychotherapists, as well as by a prevailing climate of opinion transmitted through the media. Yet it has long been known that all retrospective measures of childhood experiences have a heritable component (Plomin 1994). This reflects the fact that perceptions of life events are, at least in part, a reflection of personality traits.

Early Separation or Loss

Early separation or loss is the most factual of all risk factors and has fewer problems through distortion of memory or processing of experience. Even so, the long-term effects of losing a parent depend on many factors other than the simple facts of death or divorce (Hetherington 1993). In our own research, about half of all patients with BPD had lost a parent either through divorce or death before age 16, a quarter of them before age 5 (Paris 2020). This rate is genuinely high, because the subjects in this sample had grown up prior to the recent "epidemic" of divorce.

All things being equal, it is better to be brought up in an intact family. The obvious exceptions involve mental illness in a parent or family violence, in which case separation can even be positive for children (Rutter 1987a). However, family breakdown does not, *by itself*, create a long-term risk for psychopathology. The reason is that the effects of separation or loss from a parent during childhood depend on their interactions with other risk factors. On the whole, a pathological outcome is most likely when one negative experience leads to another, producing a "cascade" effect.

Studies of community populations of children of divorce show that, as with other childhood adversities, resilience is the rule. The problem is that although divorce does not necessarily cause a cascade, it can. Moreover, family breakdown may have a different effect, not seen in normal populations, in children who are temperamentally vulnerable.

Abnormal Parenting

Abnormal parenting is a well-supported risk factor for developing personality disorders in adulthood. Many studies have shown that patients with personality disorders are more likely to have had parents with psychiatric disorders. In BPD, parents are more likely to show personality disorders, chronic depression, or substance abuse (White et al. 2003). Although these associations could reflect common genetic vulnerabilities, it seems commonsensical to assume that living with a mentally ill parent is a stressor in its own right. Children may have a particular risk if their parent has a personality disorder, because unlike intermittent symptomatic disorders, personality pathology has a *continuous* effect on parenting capacity.

Additional evidence for the negative effects of having a parent with psychopathology comes from research on children. In recent years, the most important research project has been the Pittsburgh Girls Study (Stepp et al. 2016). A very large sample (N=2,451) of prepubertal girls was recruited and followed into adolescence. The results showed that BPD is often preceded by disruptive behavioral disorder such as ADHD and oppositional defiant disorder (Stepp et al. 2014). They also showed that traits associated with emotion dysregulation lead to high levels of family conflict, producing a vicious circle (Stepp et al. 2012).

Abnormal parenting can also be measured retrospectively through patient reports on the quality of parenting. The best-known self-report instrument for this purpose is the Parental Bonding Index (Parker 1983). This scale derives its constructs from theories of child development, which define the tasks of parenting in terms of two basic dimensions: providing affection and allowing autonomy. Research using this measure in patients with BPD (reviewed in Paris 2020) points to serious problems in bonding with parents, including both a lack of affection (neglect) and a lack of autonomy (overcontrol). However, problems in parental bonding are not very specific to any category of disorder, or even to the personality disorders as a group, and are also reported by patients with many other psychiatric diagnoses (Parker 1983).

Childhood Trauma

In converging evidence from many studies, patients with personality disorders, particularly those with BPD, often report traumatic events, particularly childhood sexual or physical abuse (Paris 2020). The problem is, little specificity exists in the relationship between trauma and BPD, and even less between trauma and personality disorders as a whole. Moreover, the effect size of this relationship in a meta-analysis of BPD was only 0.28 (Fossati et al. 1999). Therefore, even when we find a high frequency of child abuse in patients with BPD, it may not be the main cause of the disorder but only one of several risk factors.

We also need to put the relationships between trauma and personality disorders in the context of community studies of childhood sexual abuse (Browne and Finkelhor 1986) and childhood physical abuse (Malinosky-Rummell and Hansen 1993). Even though early trauma is a risk factor for a wide range of psychological symptoms in adulthood, about 80% of adults with abuse histories show no demonstrable psychopathology (Fergusson et al. 2011a, 2011b). Moreover, although the frequency of child abuse and neglect has gone down (Finkelhor et al. 1990), little change seems to have occurred in the frequency of personality disorders.

Also, community studies show that the long-term sequelae of abuse experiences depend on the severity of trauma. Most reported child abuse is of *low* severity, and this is also true in patients with personality disorders (Zanarini 2005). Unfortunately, minor incidents are sometimes scored in the same way as severe ones, leading to an inflation of the relationship. In our sample, most involved *single* incidents associated with perpetrators who are *not* family members (Paris et al. 1994).

In summary, although child abuse can be associated with pathological sequelae, the presence of abuse histories in patients fails to provide an adequate explanation of their current symptomatology. Moreover, no clinical symptoms can be used as "markers" for adversity in childhood. The effects of trauma can only be fully understood through their interactions with other risk factors and with biological predispositions. Again, the effects of *any* of the psychological stressors that are risk factors for personality disorders can be better understood in the context of interactions with biological predispositions.

A number of lines of evidence support this way of looking at the evidence. First, the association of negative events with personality disorders is partly due to common traits leading to pathological behavior in caretakers. Both diagnosable parental psychopathology and parental neglect may derive from dysfunctional personality traits that reflect a common genetic vulnerability between children and parents. Second, temperamentally difficult children are more likely to be mistreated by their families (Rutter and Quinton 1984). An irritable child is more likely to be beaten and less likely to be heard. Alternatively, parents can respond overprotectively to a child with a difficult temperament, failing to provide the limits and boundaries known to help contain impulsivity and affective instability. Third, the effects of negative events in childhood are mediated by cognitive schema. Some people have traits, such as neuroticism, that make them more vulnerable to negative events. Other, more resilient people react less strongly to life's vicissitudes and are less susceptible. Still others show differential susceptibility to the environment, responding more strongly to positive and negative influences (Rioux et al. 2018b). Any theory of the personality disorders needs to account for why different children perceive the same environment differently. In summary, traumatic experiences, however distressing, have greater impact on those who are genetically predisposed.

SOCIAL FACTORS IN THE PERSONALITY DISORDERS

The basic dimensions of personality are similar all over the world, but social expectations encourage some kinds of behavior and suppress others. Societies differ in their ability to tolerate different traits. Thus, traditional societies are more tolerant of dependence, and most individuals are expected to conform to group and family norms. On the other hand, modern societies expect high levels of autonomy, and most individuals are expected to develop their own career paths and to find their own spouses and friends (Paris 1996). These expectations are highly stressful for those who cannot easily meet them. Personality disorders should therefore have a differential prevalence across cultures.

The most solid evidence thus far concerns antisocial personality disorder, which had an increasing prevalence in North America and Europe after the Second World War (Rutter and Smith 1995). Yet antisocial personality disorder has a surprisingly low prevalence in some East Asian societies, such as Taiwan, at least when studied 30 years ago (Hwu et al. 1989). The most likely explanation is that North American families are more likely to produce the risk factors for this condition (Robins 1966). In contrast, the traditional structure of Taiwanese families and society creates a strong atmosphere of discipline and suppresses many of the impulsive behaviors in children that characterize conduct disorder.

In accordance with the observation that the most important environmental influences on personality are "unshared," the social factors in the personality disorders may depend in part on the availability of attachment figures outside the nuclear family and on access to social networks. However, children have varying capacities to make use of these networks. Social factors can be used to define an overall measure of health in the community, which has been called *social integration* (Leighton et al. 1963). In contrast, *social disintegration* is characterized by a breakdown of extended family ties, a loss of social networks, a lack of community ties, a normlessness related to the loss of consensual values, and difficulties in developing and maintaining social roles.

GENE-ENVIRONMENT MODEL OF THE PERSONALITY DISORDERS

Only a gene-environment model can account for the fact that individuals with all the psychosocial risk factors for personality disorders do not necessarily develop them, that genetic risks do not reliably predict the development of personality disorders, and that the same risks lead to different personality disorders in different people. Thus, the temperamental factors that shape personality disorders do not necessarily lead to diagnosable disorders, and psychosocial risk factors are all associated with *statistical* risks rather than with predictable effects. The relative weakness of these associations makes sense if psychosocial risks are only pathogenic in interaction with a genetic vulnerability. These observations provide support for a model in which personality disorders are the outcome of interactions between heritable traits and psychosocial risk factors. A model of this kind has been suggested by several experts on personality disorders (Beck et al. 2014; Linehan 1993; Livesley 2003).

Let us examine how we might combine the effects of biological, psychological, and social factors into this model. The biological variability in personality traits reflects temperament. However, a wide range of trait variability is compatible with normality, and trait variations are insufficient by themselves to account for the amplification of traits to disorders. On the other hand, traits are the main determinant of which type of personality disorder can develop. Thus, disorders characterized by extraversion, such as those in the impulsive cluster, do not usually develop in those who are highly introverted. Conversely, disorders characterized by introversion, such as those in the odd and anxious clusters, do not emerge in those who are highly extraverted.

Every individual has a mixture of traits: some more adaptive, others less adaptive. An unusual intensity of certain traits can lower the threshold at which stressors can trigger a personality disorder. The best example concerns the emotional instability and impulsivity that are, particularly in combination, associated with BPD.

Psychological and social factors are the crucial determinants of whether underlying traits lead to overt disorders. However, they do not by themselves *cause* personality disorders. This conclusion is supported by the evidence that most children are resilient even in the face of the most severe stressors, ranging from socioeconomic deprivation to severe parental pathology. Without temperamental vulnerability, children usually have sufficient resilience to compensate for most adversities. Personality disorders are, therefore, examples of gene-environment interactions. Some of the traits underlying personality disorders increase both *exposure* and *susceptibility* to environmental factors. Both impulsivity (associated with antisocial personality disorder) and a combination of impulsivity and affective instability (associated with BPD) are temperamental factors that make it more likely that children will be either badly treated or mishandled. Moreover, high neuroticism can make children more susceptible to stressors. These interactions between temperament and environment could play a crucial role in the pathways to impulsive disorders.

Similarly, an anxious temperament leads to social anxiety and avoidance, characteristics that interfere with peer relationships and can make children even more anxious and withdrawn. Moreover, anxious children are difficult to raise and tend to elicit either overprotection or rejection from parents. Thus, genetic factors influence both exposure and susceptibility to environmental stressors.

For most patients, the risk of developing personality pathology is greatly increased by stressful life experiences. Chronic adversities are most likely to have an amplifying effect on traits. Yet psychological protective factors consisting of positive life experiences can buffer these risk factors. Stressful experiences inside the family can also be buffered by extrafamilial attachments, which have been consistently shown to protect children at risk. The role of social factors in this model would be to influence the threshold at which traits become amplified into disorders. Social factors can be protective, such as when strong community supports buffer biological and psychological risks. Alternatively, social factors can be risks in their own right, as in the case of sociocultural disintegration.

The etiological pathways to personality disorders will be different for different diagnostic categories. Disorders in Cluster A lie in the schizophrenia spectrum and are highly heritable. Cluster B disorders derive from interactions between impulsive or affective traits and family dysfunction. Cluster C disorders derive from the amplification of anxious traits by psychosocial stressors.

CONCLUSION

Many unanswered questions remain about the etiology of the personality disorders. Most particularly, we need more longitudinal studies of children followed into adulthood to define more precisely which risk factors are most crucial. The long-held belief that personality disorders are entirely caused by childhood adversities is wrong. Their early onset and chronicity are more likely to be a reflection of temperament. Thus, the personality disorders provide one of the best exemplars of the interactions between nature and nurture.

PART III

IMPLICATIONS

CHAPTER 14

— CLINICAL IMPLICATIONS

MENTAL HEALTH clinicians aim to change patients' minds. In recent years, it has become increasingly attractive to produce change using neurochemical means. In severe mental disorders such as schizophrenia and bipolar I, that is usually the right choice. As compared with the past, modern psychiatric medications are more effective, have a wider spectrum of efficacy, and have fewer side effects. Yet patients are also people with lives that can be stressful. When clinicians apply a biopsychosocial model to treatment, they give appropriate respect to the environment of the people they treat. There are several reasons why this does not always happen. One is time and money: most insurance companies and governmental bodies have policies that encourage seeing patients for 15 minutes. Another reason is ideological: psychiatrists who believe the mantra that mental disorders are brain disorders tend to favor interventions that focus on neural systems.

The trend toward a biological orientation in psychiatry has become so pervasive that, for some practitioners, clinical work has come to consist of little but brief check-ups and the writing of prescriptions. In many settings, nonmedical mental health workers have become the primary caregivers; most psychotherapy is being provided by nonpsychiatrists. At the same time, family doctors are becoming more and more adept in psychopharmacology. The discipline of psychiatry is still struggling to define in which ways it is unique. Applying a broader model of the causes of psychopathology could help develop an alternative to this fragmentation of mental health care. Psychiatry is unique in crossing the boundaries between many disciplines. Its clinical practitioners therefore need to be *eclectic*. They also need to be committed to *evidence-based* practice, offering patients treatments that have been demonstrated to be effective in empirical research.

This chapter aims to show how a gene-environment model of psychopathology can guide clinical work. It suggests that the future of psychiatry lies in an eclectic and evidence-based practice. To show why clinical work must be integrative, I discuss the problems associated with reductionism, both biological and environmental. I illustrate these principles by examining two of the most common clinical problems in psychiatry: the treatment of major depressive disorder (MDD) and the psychotherapy of personality disorders. The point of view taken in this chapter is not unique: it has been developed by many other writers. Decades ago, Gabbard and Goodwin (1996), a psychoanalyst and a biological researcher, wrote eloquently about the value of using a stress-diathesis model to understand mental disorders, allowing practitioners to offer a broader set of treatment options. We need to put these principles into practice.

BIOLOGICAL REDUCTIONISM IN PSYCHIATRY

Reductionism is the practice of explaining complex phenomena in terms of phenomena believed to lie at a simpler or more fundamental level (Gold 2009). It contrasts with *holism*, in which the whole is seen as more than the sum of its parts and requires analysis at its own level. In principle, psychiatrists are committed to holism. Yet some of the most serious mistakes they have made in the past were based on misguided attempts to consider "the whole patient." By trying to take into account the complexity of the individual, practitioners lost sight of their responsibility to relieve distress.

Our greatest successes in therapy came in the early days of the psychopharmacological revolution. By reducing complex syndromes to targeted symptoms that respond to specific medications, psychiatrists were able to treat the most severely ill patients more effectively. In this way, reductionism has had done much good. The problem is that this approach is not really suitable for common mental disorders, such as depression and anxiety, or for complex conditions with weaker heritability, such as substance use disorders, eating disorders, and personality disorders.

I am old enough, as an undergraduate student in psychology, to have visited mental hospitals before the introduction of neuroleptics and observed the grim fate these patients once faced. Later on, first as a medical student and then as a resident, I was expected to manage a wide variety of outpatients by exploring their personal histories, without being taught any practical means to provide relief for their symptoms. Clinicians today benefit from having many more options. Over the past few decades, knowledge in the neurosciences has increased exponentially. This has dramatically changed psychiatry. Neuroscience has become a cutting edge for contemporary theory and research and the conceptual basis for developing even better forms of pharmacological treatment.

The clinical implications of these advances have been somewhat exaggerated, however. These felicitous developments have also been associated with some negative trends. For some clinicians, history taking consists of little more than a checklist used to determine whether the patient meets criteria for a DSM diagnosis. Therapy may then consist only of prescribing medications appropriate for that category. Unfortunately, this picture is not a caricature! Errors in practice are often based on misunderstandings in theory. Reductionistic models of psychopathology lead to reductionistic methods of treatment. Clinicians may forget that psychiatric diagnoses are rarely homogeneous entities. As I have argued in this book, most forms of psychopathology lie on some form of spectrum in which overt disorders emerge from complex interactions between predisposition and stressors. Moreover, similar clinical symptoms can arise from very different pathways. In some cases, predispositions will be stronger, whereas in others, the influence of the environment will be the determining factor. Clinical observations cannot separate these cases.

If each patient with the same diagnosis is different, then no simple algorithm can determine the right choice of treatment. Throughout this book, I have emphasized the importance of *individual differences*. The art of medicine also involves *individualizing* therapy. By this I do not mean "personalized medicine," in which drug treatment is guided by genetic profiles. (We are very far away from that scenario.) What I mean is taking into account a patient's life history and current environment. Good clinical practice means taking the uniqueness of every patient into account.

BEYOND REDUCTIONISM: THE TREATMENT OF MAJOR DEPRESSION

The biological revolution in psychiatry profoundly affected the treatment of MDD. It has become almost standard practice to determine whether patients meet the DSM criteria for this diagnosis and, if they do, to prescribe an antidepressant. If patients do not respond to medication, they are labeled "treatment resistant" and are offered a more complex pharmacological regimen. Yet only about half of patients have a positive response to antidepressants (Kirsch et al. 2008). These agents often have only a small advantage over placebo, and strategies such as augmentation or switching are not consistently effective for those who fail initial drug treatment (Rush et al. 2006).

Biological reductionism runs the danger of reducing patient autonomy and agency. Some people with depression may be comforted by the belief their distress is entirely due to chemical imbalances. Others use biology as an excuse to avoid dealing with life problems that should be addressed to reduce the risk of relapse. Patients with depression are heterogeneous. The most severe cases, associated with either a bipolar illness or psychotic or melancholic symptoms, have the strongest genetic predispositions. Patients with less severe depressions carry a weaker genetic load, and their illness is more influenced by environmental precipitants. Providing different treatment options for different forms of illness is therefore logical.

Moreover, the criteria for a diagnosis of MDD are very broad. Patients can meet them even when they are sleeping normally, maintaining a good appetite, and not considering suicide. To meet the criteria in DSM, it is sufficient to feel depressed most of the time, to lose interest in things, to feel excessively tired, to have difficulty concentrating, and to dislike oneself. It is far from clear that all patients meeting such criteria have the same illness. The assumption that a diagnosis of major depression, by itself, provides sufficient information to make intelligent decisions about the treatment of depression is not supported by empirical research. In fact, DSM-5 does not define any of its categories on the basis of treatment response (American Psychiatric Association 2013). With the exception of the psychoses, there is little evidence that diagnoses predict the effectiveness of *any* specific form of treatment.

Research does not support the idea that every patient with major depression *must* be treated with medications. The National Institute of Mental Health Collaborative Study of Depression (Elkin et al. 1989) found that for most patients, several forms of psychotherapy yielded equivalent results to those obtained with antidepressants. Only in severe cases, such as those with melancholia, were antidepressants clearly superior, and later studies confirmed this conclusion (Kirsch 2010). Thus, when the criteria for melancholia are absent, there is little justification to prescribe antidepressants *routinely*. Psychotherapy alone can be a perfectly adequate treatment for mild to moderate cases.

Patient preferences play a crucial role in making these clinical decisions. Some patients are only interested in pharmacotherapy for their symptoms. We can accept these preferences, given that antidepressant therapy yields positive results in a wide range of patients. However, in doing so, we need not think that we are correcting chemical imbalances. Rather, medications may act to break vicious circles, allowing patients to escape from negative feedback loops between depressed affect and depression-driven behaviors. Some patients with depression dislike taking pills, insisting that they "only want to talk." In most cases, unless depression is severe, clinicians can feel secure that psychotherapy will be effective. This is because the process of therapy, by its very nature, has a striking effect on morale (Frank and Frank 1991).

Many patients with depression prefer to receive both pharmacological and psychotherapeutic therapy. Combined treatment has the advantage of providing faster symptomatic relief while addressing the factors that lead to chronicity. This does not mean, however, that everyone needs both forms of treatment. Many patients leave treatment decisions to their therapist. Because patients often improve to a surprising degree after a single contact (Howard et al. 1986), it may be wise to hold off a decision about prescribing until the second session. If patients with nonmelancholic depression improve between the first and second contact, we will have saved them a great deal of trouble by waiting before prescribing.

The treatment of depression has to take the danger of chronicity into account. Follow-up studies show that major depression has a high rate of relapse (Shea et al. 1992). Some of this chronicity may be rooted in genetic predispositions, which can be strong enough to produce a relapse whenever drug treatment is interrupted. Alternatively, chronicity may be a result of "kindling" (see Chapter 8), in that each episode makes the next one more likely. For these reasons, a certain percentage of depressed patients need long-term pharmacological therapy.

Personality is another important factor in the chronicity of depression. Research following up treated patients demonstrates that *any* personality disorder comorbidity makes it much less likely that drug therapy will be successful in managing depressive symptoms (Shea et al. 1989). Moreover, such comorbidity is far from uncommon: research finds that most patients with personality disorders are depressed and that up to half of depressed patients also have a personality disorder (Friborg et al. 2014). These findings have important clinical implications.

An important subgroup (perhaps the majority) of depressed patients need treatment beyond the prescription of pharmacotherapy. They are not just "treatment resistant" to medications but do not respond to them and need psychotherapy. This is why recent clinical guidelines for the treatment of borderline personality disorder (BPD) do *not* recommend the prescription of antidepressants (National Institute for Health and Care Excellence 2015).

Some clinicians seem to have forgotten that depression is rooted in personality. This insight was long a defining concept in psychiatry and helps us to see each patient as a person and to take into account important individual differences that go beyond diagnosis. Moreover, if changing medications is all we do, we miss other significant factors maintaining depressed mood. By failing to take the time to make a systematic assessment of personality, clinicians reduce their ability to predict which patients are most likely to benefit from symptomatic treatment. Even in schizophrenia, a disorder known to be strongly biological, rehabilitative psychosocial interventions markedly reduce the risk of relapse (Turkington et al. 2004).

Diagnoses in psychiatry are useful modes for communication but need not be thought of as "real" entities. Categorizing patients can provide an overall guideline to understanding them but is usually insufficient for making a detailed treatment plan. It was only when biological psychiatry became the dominant paradigm in psychiatry that specific and well-defined criteria became a practical possibility. To provide a comprehensive assessment of cases, DSM devised a complex system with five axes. The problem was, clinicians often only used one axis, the one that describes symptoms. In the end, the five-axis system was dropped in DSM-5.

Many clinicians are satisfied once they make a symptomatic diagnosis. The reason is the wish to identify conditions that are treatable with medication. Even if the assumption that making a symptomatic diagnosis is sufficient were true (and it often is *not*), this approach to practice ignores the mediating factors measured on the other axes: personality, stressors, and functional level. The result of one-dimensional diagnosis is one-dimensional therapy.

ENVIRONMENTAL REDUCTIONISM IN PSYCHIATRY

Environmental reductionism is usually associated with the practice of psychotherapy. Psychotherapists may favor these theories because they seem to provide a more hopeful prognosis. If the primary roots of psychological symptoms lie in childhood, then symptoms might be reversed if negative experiences are addressed in treatment. If psychopathology is simply the result of learning the wrong thing, or having the wrong parents, then providing a new point of view might reverse these effects.

Some psychotherapists resist genetic theories of mental illness on the grounds that heredity implies irreversibility. That conclusion is based on a series of misunderstandings. First, the mechanisms by which genes affect the mind are complex and indirect. Second, genetic influences on behavior are never independent of the environment. Third, people with problematic heritable traits can change, and talking therapy can help them to do so. This is clearly the case for BPD, which is usually treatable with psychotherapy (Paris 2020).

Moreover, even when the variance in a trait is entirely a function of genes, it can still be modified by environmental factors. A famous example is phenylketonuria. This inborn error of metabolism causes serious illness beginning at birth that, if untreated, leads inevitably to severe mental retardation. Yet, although the etiology of this disease is entirely due to a defect on a single gene, it can be treated successfully by a simple alteration in diet. Patients who follow this diet go on to live a completely normal life. This example demonstrates that focusing on genetic factors in psychopathology need not lead to therapeutic nihilism or to the downgrading of psychotherapy.

Psychotherapists may also be suspicious of genetic constraints on individual development because they contradict a cherished belief in the unlimited nature of human potential. In contrast, a gene-environment model suggests a rather different treatment philosophy. It encourages therapists to be more modest in their expectations. It is concordant with a world view in which people need to learn to accept the limits of the human condition.

Finally, psychotherapists may be reluctant to consider the predispositions to mental disorders if they believe that doing so involves "blaming the victim." Unfortunately, this line of thought implies that there *is* a victim. Of course, parents *do* make serious mistakes when raising their children, and some life events *do* lie outside our control. But if one seeks recovery, one needs *agency*—the feeling of being in charge of one's own life.

Individuals vary widely in their response to negative events. This fact need not be used to support the conclusion that patients are responsible for their own difficulties. By taking both nature and nurture into account, we can avoid attributions of blame. Psychotherapists need to take individual differences into account. When the tailor has only one size, the customer must pay for the adjustments. One of the strengths of the gene-environment model is that it addresses individuality while leaving sufficient space for personal responsibility and existential choice. If personality is often the main factor determining how individuals respond to life's challenges, then therapy must be conducted differently with different people.

In the future, psychological treatments will be based on more interactive etiological theories. "Dynamic formulations" of psychopathology fail to take into account how the same experiences have different effects on individuals with different personality traits. Personality disorders provide an example of how this principle can be applied in practice.

BEYOND REDUCTIONISM: THE TREATMENT OF PERSONALITY DISORDERS

In recent years, the province of the psychotherapist has been shrinking. Although most therapy in practice is brief, many believe that long-term difficulties must require long-term treatments. Clinical tradition has considered open-ended therapy to be the treatment of choice for personality disorders, but this kind of therapy is very expensive and inaccessible for most people. Moreover, this perception acts a barrier to briefer treatments that have been shown to be efficacious. There is also little evidence that long-term treatments for personality disorders are effective.

Given their reputation for being hard to treat, patients with personality disorders have long been unpopular among psychiatrists (Lewis and Appleby 1988). If they can afford it, however, these patients may still be offered long-term psychotherapy. Up to recently, such methods have been based on the assumption of the primacy of early experience. These theories all encourage therapists to explore the events of childhood in great detail. Yet there can be negative effects associated with methods that relate problems in the present primarily to events in the past. Patients can use childhood experiences to validate their sense of victimization or to rationalize avoiding change. Therapists may also become embroiled in the process of gaining "insight" and lose sight of problems that need to be addressed in the present. Finally, psychotherapy that holds parents accountable for their children's difficulties runs the risk of depriving patients of needed support from family members. This set of problems would be less likely to arise if therapists based their treatments on a gene-environment model. Doing so would allow them to have reasonable expectations for change and to focus on solving problems in the present rather than allowing people to ruminate about the past.

We now have more precise and better supported methods of psychotherapy for personality disorders. The most widely used treatment is dialectical behavior therapy for BPD (Linehan 1993). Several evidence-based alternatives can be shortened to make them less expensive and more accessible (Paris 2020). All current methods help patients regulate their emotions, avoid impulsive actions, and have better strategies to deal with relationships. Taking this highly practical point of view, patients with personality disorders can often be treated quite rapidly (Paris 2017).

Because genetic factors are involved in the etiology of personality disorders, we will eventually need to develop methods of treatment that address the role of heritable traits. For now, however, medications are, at best, of marginal value for this patient population (National Institute for Health and Care Excellence 2015). Instead, psychotherapists can work with traits, which, even if grounded in biological variations, have been amplified by social learning. Psychotherapy, a new form of social learning, aims to reverse this process. In dialectical behavior therapy (Linehan 1993), impulsivity and affective instability are reduced by psychoeducational methods that target these traits, teaching patients how to tolerate dysphoric emotions.

No matter what the theory, the ultimate goal of any psychotherapy has to be behavioral modification. Traits express themselves through behavior and must therefore be modified through an educational process requiring patients to practice new behaviors in their daily lives. This means that patients have to start changing early in the treatment. This could involve "getting a life" through work or school or ending toxic relationships and finding better ones. Change also involves knowing one's personality and learning to capitalize on it.

Psychotherapy in the personality disorders therefore requires integrating multiple perspectives. One needs to take into account the historical circumstances that originally led to trait amplification and continue to affect perceptions of current relationships. Understanding life experiences also provides empathy, communicating the therapist's interest in the patient as a person. Moreover, knowing the historical origins of maladaptive behavior patterns can be useful in demonstrating that they are being anachronistically applied to present situations.

It should be kept in mind that explaining behavior is rarely a sine qua non for change. History is only a first step. As every therapist knows, patients are often at a loss as to how to apply self-knowledge they gain from treatment. Patients must learn how to modify traits through behavioral change. This usually requires intensive practice in the laboratory of the patient's current interpersonal relationships. Most of the work for the therapist involves focusing on maladaptive patterns in the patient's *present* life, working with the patient to develop adaptive alternatives. Yet understanding can only be complete when we take predispositions into account. Blaming the past creates "narratives" that either are not true or are misleading justification for victimhood. Instead, patients need to know that they differ in their sensitivities and that different people process experience in different ways. Therapists applying this approach can describe a patient's temperament, explain how traits interacted with life experiences, and show how amplification eventually created difficulties in the patient's present life.

Let us consider some examples. A patient with an impulsive temperament might be told, "Given your active way of dealing with problems, you do not always understand what you are feeling inside, making it particularly hard for you to deal with what happens to you. What makes this even harder is that you had no one to show you how to deal with your emotions. Even now, you find upset feelings difficult and often end up doing things you regret instead of looking first at how you feel inside and then figuring out a way to solve a problem." Similarly, anxious people who are introverted or "slow to warm up" tend to become more withdrawn when stressed, as in avoidant personality disorder. A patient with anxious traits might be told, "Because of your natural shyness, you are particularly sensitive to rejection and withdraw even further. What makes this even harder was that you had no one who could help you master these feelings. Even now, you often end up avoiding situations that scare you instead of accepting feelings and learning how to get past them."

The idea of using temperament in psychotherapy is not new. Decades ago, Burks and Rubenstein (1979) recommended giving patients a temperament scale to help them understand their vulnerabilities. However, we probably need to know a great deal more about the biological nature of personality traits before making them the basis of a systematic approach to psychotherapy.

Cognitive-behavioral therapy is the only form of psychological therapy that consistently uses a gene-environment model of psychopathology. For example, Beck (1979) conceptualized depression as resulting from interactions between a heritable predisposition to lowered mood and life experiences that produced hopelessness and helplessness. Beck et al. (2014) later developed a similar model to account for and to treat personality disorders.

Linehan's (1993) treatment model for BPD is also based on a predisposition-stress (or gene-environment) theory. Linehan hypothesizes that patients with BPD begin life with a predisposition to emotional dysregulation. Negative experiences, which Linehan terms an "invalidating environment," increase this instability to pathological proportions. The treatment of BPD therefore consists of psychoeducational methods that help these patients regulate their emotions so that they can learn how to solve interpersonal problems. This approach may well turn out to be a model for the treatment of many forms of mental disorder.

CONCLUSION

The relationship between nature and nurture provides the conceptual basis for an eclectic clinical practice. The most important principle is that different patients with the same diagnosis require different forms of treatment. Patients are most likely to require biological interventions when their predispositions are so strong that even the mildest of stressors overwhelm them. This is often the case for most patients with schizophrenia and with severe mood disorders. In patients with milder predispositions, multiple stressors can produce symptoms by overwhelming resilience. This is often the case for most patients with mild depressions and anxiety disorders.

Treating symptoms with pharmacological interventions often hastens recovery and allows normal coping mechanisms to be reinstituted. However, many patients with depression or anxiety can be treated effectively with psychotherapy alone. Ideally, we should offer our patients the facts and give them the choice. In most cases, combined methods of treatment are the best way to address predisposing and stressing factors in psychopathology. In this respect, being a medical practitioner has some advantage, because the same clinician can offer both psychopharmacology and psychotherapy.

Clinicians should never prescribe medication mechanically but consider the life stressors, as well as the personality traits, that elicit and maintain symptoms. Similarly, when we prescribe psychotherapy, we can frame the patient's history against a background of individual differences in temperament and personality. Understanding personality traits can be crucial in the prevention of chronicity. Finally, a predisposition-stress model leads to a different *philosophy* of treatment. When clinicians take predispositions into account, their goals for patients are much more likely to be pragmatic.

CHAPTER 15

IMPLICATIONS FOR PREVENTION AND FURTHER RESEARCH

NATURE, NURTURE, AND PREVENTION

Clinicians have always been interested in interventions to protect people against mental illness before it starts. However, in order to develop a rational strategy for prevention, we would need accurate etiological models of the illnesses we hope to prevent. In the 1960s, there was a great burst of enthusiasm for the concept of a preventive psychiatry. Unfortunately, the ideas behind the community psychiatry movement were based on strong environmental assumptions. For example, Caplan (1961) suggested that providing children with a better psychological and social environment could prevent a wide range of adult mental disorders. Unfortunately, these beliefs were based on faith, not facts. Thus far, little solid empirical evidence has shown that mental disorders can be effectively prevented through psychosocial interventions.

Today, hope for prevention is more likely to be based on neurobiology and genetics. The idea that early intervention and personalized medicine will revolutionize our approach to severe mental disorders offers hope but has yet to be supported by evidence. We have more psychiatrists, more clinical psychologists, and more mental health workers of every kind than at any other point in human history, yet mental disorders are hardly less common. In the postwar era (Kessler et al. 2005; Robins and Regier 1991), several important conditions: depression, substance abuse, and antisocial personality, became *more* prevalent than they were a few decades previously.

The most likely explanation for increases in the prevalence of depression, substance abuse, and antisocial personality derives from social stressors. Clinicians have no control over these risk factors, most of which are derived from profound forces that are disrupting the family and community ties that once provided people with a sense of identity (Paris 1996). Only the most grandiose therapist could believe that mental health workers can provide anything but very minimal bulwarks and buffers to counter the juggernaut of modernity.

Past efforts at prevention were also based on an incorrect model of the etiology of mental illness. Environmental theories failed to take genetic factors into account, and genetic theories failed to take the environment into account. A preventive psychiatry grounded in a gene-environment model of psychopathology could avoid repeating the naïve optimism of the past. A crucial aspect of prevention in the future could involve developing the means to identify biological predispositions prior to the onset of mental disorders. Medicine is on the verge of being able to determine profiles that could define the genetic vulnerability to disease in each individual. Some fear that this information might only frighten and demoralize people.

This need not be the case. For example, if we know we are genetically prone to coronary artery disease, we can take particular care of our diet, exercise, and avoid smoking. Similarly, if we know we are prone to either essential hypertension or type II diabetes mellitus, we can take action to minimize our risk. Even if we know that we are *not* prone to any of these diseases, we do not have the freedom to lead a totally unhealthy lifestyle, because longevity itself depends on the same environmental risk factors. Although we cannot avoid falling ill, we can, at the very least, save ourselves a great deal of trouble.

How might we apply these principles to psychiatry? The first step involves accurate measurements of the predispositions to illness. We already do this, in a rough fashion, by determining whether patients have a family history of a disease. In the future, we can become more precise by carrying out specific biological tests to determine whether an unaffected individual is vulnerable to illness. Moreover, taking into account the polygenic nature of most psychiatric illness, we can determine the *quantitative* strength of that predisposition.

These tests will almost certainly involve measurements of biological markers. In 50 years, patients going to psychiatrists will probably be expected to have routine bloodwork. In addition, some of the "high-tech" procedures of today, such as imaging, could eventually become accessible for office practitioners. In spite of the disappointments following the decoding of the genome, it might in principle provide sufficient information to *change* genetic predispositions. Gene therapy for mental disorders may sound like science fiction but is probably an inevitable development that will become a practical reality sometime in the future (and by "the future," I do not mean the next 5–10 years but by end of the twenty-first century).

In the meantime, genetic information can be used to modify environmental factors, preventing the *expression* of genetic predispositions. For example, the sons of fathers with alcoholism are an important target group for early education aimed at preventing them from abusing alcohol or other substances. Similarly, individuals prone to depression could be an important target population for preventive psychotherapy. Therapists treating this group would carry out psychological interventions designed to teach patients to buffer the influence of stressors and to improve the quality of their lives, thus reducing their overall risk for depression.

Disorders arising primarily from biological factors might also be the target of preventive strategies. At present, we have few markers for any of these diseases. However, there might be practical advantages if we could identify genetic risks early enough. In the case of schizophrenia, many groups are working on the management of early psychosis, but the risk might need to be identified as early as fetal life, because some of the environmental risk factors for this disease develop occur prior to birth. On the other hand, if we knew who was vulnerable to the illness, we could at least offer them faster treatment.

One mental disorder about which we have a great deal of genetic information is Alzheimer's disease. Evidence has shown that a specific gene producing apolipoprotein E has a polymorphism that is present in about 70% of those who eventually develop the disease (Liu et al. 2013). One might think that, given the prognosis of Alzheimer's disease, people would not want to know about their predispositions. However, that would change if treatment became a practical reality.

In summary, an effective strategy for prevention in psychiatry would require identifying vulnerable individuals and then targeting any interventions to reach individuals and populations at greatest risk. We are many decades away from this kind of knowledge.

APPLYING A GENE-ENVIRONMENT MODEL TO ETIOLOGICAL RESEARCH

Mental disorders arise from a combination of genetic vulnerability and environmental factors. Research should aim to determine their relative contributions, as well as the interactions between them, in every form of psychiatric illness. Yet when we read the literature, we rarely find investigations looking at nature and nurture in the same patients. By and large, genetic studies confine themselves to biological factors, and environmental studies confine themselves to psychosocial factors.

The problem is that we cannot usually control for the effects of genetic factors when we study environmental risks, and we cannot easily control for the effects of environmental variability when we study genetic risks. The development of genetic epidemiology could bridge this gap. Thus far, much of the research in this discipline depends on twin studies, which are limited either to traits in normal populations or to disorders with a high enough prevalence to produce sufficient numbers of affected pairs.

At present, even in well-researched diagnoses such as schizophrenia, we have no markers to determine precise levels of genetic vulnerability. We must still make use of cruder measures, such as the presence of positive family histories. Yet even within these limitations, we could develop research strategies to take gene-environment interactions into account. For example, in studying mood disorders, research should determine whether life stresses are more likely to lead to depression in those with a family history of mood disorder or less likely to do so in those without such a history.

Research on the causes of the mental disorders should therefore be *multivariate*. The statistical methods of measuring multivariate relationships are widely known, as shown by the frequency of papers in current journals using regression analyses. These methods allow us to study the percentage of the variance in any disorder accounted for by biological and psychosocial etiological factors. Moreover, research measuring predispositions and stressors in the same samples could help us overcome the misleading impressions created by univariate associations between risk factors and illness. As long as studies measure genetic or environmental factors separately, we are more easily tempted to read their findings as explanations rather than associations. Studies that examine genetic and environmental factors in the same research design would need to use sophisticated methods of assessment. Including a measure of "trauma" in a biological study or a single genetic polymorphism in a study of environmental effects is not good enough.

Finally, research on nature and nurture in psychiatry could help us to develop a new and better system of classifying mental disorders. Ultimately, psychiatric diagnoses will be based on common predispositions, and measures of stress will remain important as a way of accounting for thresholds of liability for illness.

CONCLUSIONS: INTEGRATING NATURE AND NURTURE

I have written this book to offer clinicians a better and more comprehensive model of the probable causes of mental illness. The theory presented here is only a first step toward addressing the question posed in the introduction: why, in the presence of the same environmental challenges, do some people develop one type of disorder while others develop an entirely different type? At our present state of knowledge, this book can only provide a brief sketch of an answer to this question. However, given the present pace and trajectory of psychiatric research, we can expect that the next few decades will yield data to fill in the picture in greater detail. We are just beginning to understand the genetic factors in mental disorders. The study of environmental risk factors is also at an early stage.

Therefore, many of the details described in this book are sure to change. The more successful research is, the more likely will it be that many of the conclusions presented here will become obsolete. What will probably *not* change, however, is the basic principle that most mental disorders have a genetic component and that environmental factors uncover these underlying vulnerabilities. Psychiatric theory is undergoing a transition, paralleling changes in other disciplines seeking to understand human behavior. Eventually, the pendulum swing between nature and nurture will be less wild. With time, gene-environment interactions will become the normal frame for thinking about psychopathology. With time, ideas that once seemed overly complex will become truisms.

One word of warning is necessary. Social scientists and mental health workers have long predicted the imminent demise of the nature-nurture dichotomy. In principle, most clinicians have long accepted that "either/or" has to be replaced by "both together." Yet the split between nature and nurture continues. The political, social, and emotional implications of this debate have led many scientists and clinicians to take one side and ignore the other. A strong commitment to empirical methods in psychiatry could help to counteract these "gut reactions." The ultimate truth concerning scientific questions need not depend on their practical implications. We must be dispassionate about the truth. Science tells us that nature cannot be understood without nurture, and that nurture cannot be understood without nature. We need to listen to this message, and make it an integral part of our practice.

REFERENCES

Agnew-Blais JC, Polanczyk GV, Danese A, et al: Evaluation of the persistence, remission, and emergence of attention-deficit/hyperactivity disorder in young adulthood. JAMA Psychiatry 73(7):713–720, 2016

Allen KL, Gibson LY, McLean NJ, et al: Maternal and family factors and child eating pathology: risk and protective relationships. J Eat Disord 2:11, 2014

Alnaes R, Torgersen S: Personality and personality disorders predict development and relapses of major depression. Acta Psychiatr Scand 95(4):336–342, 1997

Amato PR, Booth A: A Generation at Risk: Growing Up in an Era of Family Upheaval. Cambridge, MA, Harvard University Press, 1997

American Psychiatric Association: Diagnostic and Statistical Manual of Mental Disorders. Washington, DC, American Psychiatric Association, 1952

American Psychiatric Association: Diagnostic and Statistical Manual of Mental Disorders, 2nd Edition. Washington, DC, American Psychiatric Association, 1968

American Psychiatric Association: Diagnostic and Statistical Manual of Mental Disorders, 3rd Edition. Washington, DC, American Psychiatric Association, 1980

American Psychiatric Association: Diagnostic and Statistical Manual of Mental Disorders, 5th Edition. Arlington, VA, American Psychiatric Association, 2013

Arribas-Ayllon M, Bartlett A, Lewis J: Psychiatric Genetics: From Hereditary Madness to Big Biology. New York, Routledge, 2019

Bagot RC, Zhang T-Y, Wen X, et al: Variations in postnatal maternal care and the epigenetic regulation of metabotropic glutamate receptor 1 expression and hippocampal function in the rat. Proc Nat Acad Sci 109 (suppl 2):17200–17207, 2012

Baker JH, Schaumberg K, Munn-Chernoff MA: Genetics of anorexia nervosa. Curr Psychiatry Rep 19(11):84, 2017

Bandura A: Self-efficacy: toward a unifying theory of behavioral change. Psychol Rev 84(2):191–215, 1977

Barch DM: Resting-state functional connectivity in the Human Connectome Project: current status and relevance to understanding psychopathology. Harv Rev Psychiatry 25(5):209–217, 2017

Barkley R (ed): Attention-Deficit Hyperactivity Disorder: A Handbook for Diagnosis and Treatment, 4th Edition. New York, Guilford, 2014

Beck AT: Cognitive Therapy and the Emotional Disorders. New York, Penguin, 1979

Beck AT, Davis DD, Freeman A: Cognitive Therapy of Personality Disorders, 3rd Edition. New York, Guilford, 2014

Belsky J, Pluess M: The nature (and nurture?) of plasticity in early human development. Perspect Psychol Sci 4(4):345–351, 2009

Bentall RP: Doctoring the Mind: Is Our Current Treatment of Mental Illness Really Any Good? New York, New York University Press, 2009

Bergen SE, Petryshen TL: Genome-wide association studies (GWAS) of schizophrenia: does bigger lead to better results? Curr Opin Psychiatry 25(2):76–82, 2012

Berrios GE: History of the affective disorders, in Handbook of Affective Disorders, 2nd Edition. Edited by Paykel ES. New York, Guilford, 1992, pp 43–56

Biederman J, Milberger S, Faraone SV, et al: Family environment risk factors for attention-deficit hyperactivity disorder: a test of Rutter's indicators of adversity. Arch Gen Psychiatry 52(6):464–470, 1995

Biederman J, Faraone S, Milberger S, et al: Predictors of persistence and remission of ADHD into adolescence: results from a four-year prospective follow-up study. J Am Acad Child Adolesc Psychiatry 35(3):343–351, 1996

Bierut LJ: Genetic vulnerability and susceptibility to substance dependence. Neuron 69(4):618–627, 2011

Bilder RM: Neuropsychology and neurophysiology in schizophrenia. Curr Opin Psychiatry 9:57–62, 1996

Binder EB: Polygenic risk scores in schizophrenia: ready for the real world? Am J Psychiatry 176(10):783–784, 2019

Birur B, Kraguljac NV, Shelton RC, Lahti AC: Brain structure, function, and neurochemistry in schizophrenia and bipolar disorder—a systematic review of the magnetic resonance neuroimaging literature. NPJ Schizophr 3:15, 2017

Black DW, Noyes R Jr, Pfohl B, et al: Personality disorder in obsessive-compulsive volunteers, well comparison subjects, and their first-degree relatives. Am J Psychiatry 150(8):1226–1232, 1993

Black DW, Gunter T, Loveless P, et al: Antisocial personality disorder in incarcerated offenders: psychiatric comorbidity and quality of life. Ann Clin Psychiatry 22(2):113–120, 2010

Blashfield R, Noyes R, Reich J, et al: Personality disorder traits in generalized anxiety and panic disorder patients. Compr Psychiatry 35(5):329–334, 1994

Boksa P: Abnormal synaptic pruning in schizophrenia: urban myth or reality? J Psychiatry Neurosci 37(2):75–77, 2012

Border R, Johnson EC, Evans LM, et al: No support for historical candidate gene or candidate gene-by-interaction hypotheses for major depression across multiple large samples. Am J Psychiatry 176(5):376–387, 2019

Bornovalova MA, Hicks BM, Iacono WG, McGue M: Stability, change, and heritability of borderline personality disorder traits from adolescence to adulthood: a longitudinal twin study. Dev Psychopathol 21(4):1335–1353, 2009

Bornovalova MA, Hicks BM, Iacono WG, McGue M: Longitudinal twin study of borderline personality disorder traits and substance use in adolescence: developmental change, reciprocal effects, and genetic and environmental influences. Personal Disord 4(1):23–32, 2013

Bornstein MH, Putnick DL, Gartstein MA, et al: Infant temperament: stability by age, gender, birth order, term status, and socioeconomic status. Child Dev 86(3):844–863, 2015

Borsboom D, Cramer AOJ, Kalis A: Brain disorders? Not really: why network structures block reductionism in psychopathology research. Behav Brain Sci 42(e2):1–54, 2019

Bowlby J: Attachment and Loss, Vol 3: Loss, Sadness and Depression. New York, Basic Books, 1980

Boyce WT: The Orchid and the Dandelion: Why Some Children Struggle and How All Can Thrive. New York, Penguin, 2019

Brenner MH: Mental Illness and the Economy. Cambridge MA, Harvard University Press, 1973

Breslau N, Davis GC, Andreski P, Peterson E: Traumatic events and posttraumatic stress disorder in an urban population of young adults. Arch Gen Psychiatry 48(3):216–222, 1991

Brown GW, Harris T: Social Origins of Depression: A Study of Psychiatric Disorder in Women. New York, Free Press, 1978

Brown GW, Harris TO, Hepworth C: Life events and endogenous depression: a puzzle re-examined. Arch Gen Psychiatry 51(7):525–534, 1994

Browne A, Finkelhor D: Impact of child sexual abuse: a review of the literature. Psychol Bull 99(1):66–77, 1986

Brumberg JJ: Fasting Girls: The Emergence of Anorexia Nervosa as a Modern Disease. Cambridge MA, Harvard University Press, 1988

Brune M: Textbook of Evolutionary Psychiatry and Psychosomatic Medicine: The Origins of Psychopathology. New York, Oxford University Press, 2015

Bryant RA: Post-traumatic stress disorder: a state-of-the-art review of evidence and challenges. World Psychiatry 18(3):259–269, 2019

Bulik CM, Sullivan PF, Wade TD, Kendler KS: Twin studies of eating disorders: a review. Int J Eat Disord 27(1):1–20, 2000

Burks J, Rubenstein M: Temperament Styles in Adult Interaction: Applications in Psychotherapy. New York, Brunner/Mazel, 1979

Bush WS, Moore JH: Chapter 11: genome-wide association studies. PLoS Comput Biol 8(12):e1002822, 2012

Buss D (ed): Evolutionary Psychology: The New Science of the Mind, 6th Edition. New York, Routledge, 2019

Buydens-Branchey L, Branchey MH, Noumair D: Age of alcoholism onset, I: relationship to psychopathology. Arch Gen Psychiatry 46(3):225–230, 1989

Byrd AL, Manuck SB: MAOA, childhood maltreatment, and antisocial behavior: meta-analysis of a gene-environment interaction. Biol Psychiatry 75(1):9–17, 2014

Cadoret RJ, Yates WR, Troughton E, et al: Genetic-environmental interaction in the genesis of aggressivity and conduct disorders. Arch Gen Psychiatry 52(11):916–924, 1995

Cantor-Graae E, Selten JP: Schizophrenia and migration: a meta-analysis and review. Am J Psychiatry 162(1):12–24, 2005

Canuso CM, Pandina G: Gender and schizophrenia. Psychopharmacol Bull 40(4):178–190, 2007

Caplan G: Prevention of Mental Disorders in Children. New York, Basic Books, 1961

Carbonneau R, Vitaro F, Tremblay RE: School adjustment and substance use in early adolescent boys: association with paternal alcoholism with and without dad in the home. Journal of Early Adolescence 38(7):1008–1035, 2018

Carey N: Junk DNA: A Journey Through the Dark Matter of the Genome. New York, Columbia University Press, 2015

Caspi A, Moffitt TE: All for one and one for all: mental disorders in one dimension. Am J Psychiatry 175(9):831–844, 2018

Caspi A, Moffitt TE, Newman DL, Silva PA: Behavioral observations at age 3 years predict adult psychiatric disorders: longitudinal evidence from a birth cohort. Arch Gen Psychiatry 53(11):1033–1039, 1996

Caspi A, McClay J, Moffitt TE, et al: Role of genotype in the cycle of violence in maltreated children. Science 297(5582):851–854, 2002

Caspi A, Sugden K, Moffitt TE, et al: Influence of life stress on depression: moderation by a polymorphism in the 5-HTT gene. Science 301(5631):386–389, 2003

Caspi A, Houts RM, Belsky DW, et al: The p factor: one general psychopathology factor in the structure of psychiatric disorders? Clin Psychol Sci 2(2):119–137, 2014

Cassidy J, Shaver PR: Handbook of Attachment: Theory, Research, and Clinical Applications, 3rd Edition. New York, Guilford, 2016

Chess S, Thomas A: Origins and Evolution of Behavior Disorders. New York, Brunner/Mazel, 1984

Childs B, Scriver CR: Age at onset and causes of disease. Perspect Biol Med 29(3 Pt 1):437–460, 1986

Childs B, Moxon ER, Winkelstein JA: Genetics and infectious disease, in The Genetic Basis of Common Diseases. Edited by King RA, Rotter JI, Motulsky AG. New York, Oxford University Press, 1992, pp 71–91

Cicchetti D: Developmental Psychopathology, 3rd Edition. New York, Wiley, 2016

Cicchetti D, Rogosch FA: Equifinality and multifinality in developmental psychopathology. Dev Psychopathol 8(4):597–600, 1996

Cicchetti D, Rogosch FA, Thibodeau EL: The effects of child maltreatment on early signs of antisocial behavior: genetic moderation by tryptophan hydroxylase, serotonin transporter, and monoamine oxidase A genes. Dev Psychopathol 24(3):907–928, 2012

Clarke AM, Clarke ADB: Early Experience: Myth and Evidence. New York, Free Press, 1979

Clarke TH, Adams MJ, Davies G: Genome-wide association study of alcohol consumption and genetic overlap with other health-related traits in UK Biobank (N=112 117). Mol Psychiatry 22(10):1376–1384, 2017

Cloninger CR: A systematic method for clinical description and classification of personality variants: a proposal. Arch Gen Psychiatry 44(6):573–588, 1987

Coelewij L, Curtis D: Mini-review: update on the genetics of schizophrenia. Ann Hum Genet 82(5):239–243, 2018

Cohen P, Crawford TN, Johnson JG, Kasen S: The Children in the Community Study of developmental course of personality disorder. J Pers Disord 19(5):466–486, 2005

Cohen JR, Menon SV, Shorey RC, et al: The distal consequences of physical and emotional neglect in emerging adults: a person-centered, multi-wave, longitudinal study. Child Abuse Negl 63:151–161, 2017

Colizzi M, Murray R: Cannabis and psychosis: what do we know and what should we do? Brit J Psychiatry 212(4):195–196, 2018

Connelly R, Platt L: Cohort profile: UK Millennium Cohort Study (MCS). Int J Epidemiol 43(6):1719–1725, 2014

Conners CK: Conners Comprehensive Behavior Rating Scales Manual. Toronto, ON, Canada, Multi-Health Systems, 2008

CorfieldEC, Yang Y, Martin NG, Nyholt DR: A continuum of genetic liability for minor and major depression. Transl Psychiatry 7(5):e1131, 2017

Corning PA: The re-emergence of "emergence": a venerable concept in search of a theory. Complexity 7(6):18–30, 2002

Cortese S, Kelly C, Chabernaud C, et al: Toward systems neuroscience of ADHD: a meta-analysis of 55 fMRI studies. Am J Psychiatry 169(10):1038–1055, 2012

Costello EJ, Erkanli A, Angold A: Is there an epidemic of child or adolescent depression? J Child Psychol Psychiatry 47(12):1263–1271, 2006

Costello EJ, Copeland W, Angold A: The Great Smoky Mountains Study: developmental epidemiology in the southeastern United States. Soc Psychiatry Psychiatr Epidemiol 51(5):639–646, 2016

Coyne JC, Whiffen VE: Issues in personality as diathesis for depression: the case of sociotropy-dependency and autonomy–self-criticism. Psychol Bull 118(3):358–378, 1995

Craddock N, Owen MJ: The beginning of the end for the Kraepelinian dichotomy. Br J Psychiatry 186:364–366, 2005

Craddock N, O'Donovan MC, Owen MJ: Genes for schizophrenia and bipolar disorder? Implications for psychiatric nosology. Schizophr Bull 32(1):9–16, 2006

Cronin H: The Ant and the Peacock: Altruism and Sexual Selection From Darwin to Today. Cambridge, UK, Cambridge University Press, 1991

Cross-Disorder Group of the Psychiatric Genomics Consortium: Genomic relationships, novel loci, and pleiotropic mechanisms across eight psychiatric disorders. Cell 179(7):1469.e11–1482.e11, 2019

Crowell SE, Beauchaine TP, Linehan MM: A biosocial developmental model of borderline personality: elaborating and extending Linehan's theory. Psychol Bull 135(3):495–510, 2009

Culverhouse RC, Saccone NL, Horton AC, et al: Collaborative meta-analysis finds no evidence of a strong interaction between stress and 5-HTTLPR genotype contributing to the development of depression. Mol Psychiatry 23(1):133–142, 2018

Cuthbert BN, Insel TR: Toward the future of psychiatric diagnosis: the seven pillars of RDoC. BMC Med 11:126, 2013

Dahlenburg SC, Gleaves DH, Hutchinson AD: Anorexia nervosa and perfectionism: a meta-analysis. Int J Eat Disord 52(3):219–229, 2019

Davies MN, Verdi S, Burri A: Generalised anxiety disorder—a twin study of genetic architecture, genome-wide association and differential gene expression. PLoS One 10(8):e0134865, 2015

Dean M, Carrington M, Winkler C, et al: Genetic restriction of HIV-1 infection and progression to AIDS by a deletion allele of the CKR5 structural gene:

Hemophilia Growth and Development Study, Multicenter AIDS Cohort Study, Multicenter Hemophilia Cohort Study, San Francisco City Cohort, ALIVE Study. Science 273(5283):1856–1862, 1996

Demontis D, Walters RK, Martin J, et al: Discovery of the first genome-wide significant risk loci for attention deficit/hyperactivity disorder. Nat Genet 51(1):63–75, 2019

Dick DM, Aliev F, Krueger RF, et al: Genome-wide association study of conduct disorder symptomatology. Mol Psychiatry 16(8):800–808, 2011

DiNicola VF: Anorexia multiforme: self-starvation in historical and cultural context, part I: self-starvation as a historical chameleon. Transcultural Psychiatric Research Review 27(3):165–196, 1990

DiRago AC, Vaillant GE: Resilience in inner city youth: childhood predictors of occupational status across the lifespan. J Youth Adolesc 36:61–70, 2007

Distel MA, Trull TJ, Derom CA, et al: Heritability of borderline personality disorder features is similar across three countries. Psychol Med 38(9):1219–1229, 2008

Dobkin PL, Tremblay RE, Sacchitelle C: Predicting boys' early-onset substance abuse from father's alcoholism, son's disruptiveness, and mother's parenting behavior. J Consult Clin Psychol 65(1):86–92, 1997

Dodge KA: Mechanisms of gene-environment interaction effects in the development of conduct disorder. Perspect Psychol Sci 4(4):408–414, 2009

Dohrenwend BP, Turse N, Yager T, Wall M: Surviving Vietnam: Psychological Consequences of the War for U.S. Veterans. New York, Oxford University Press, 2019

Duncan L, Ratanatharathorn A, Aiello AE, et al: Largest GWAS of PTSD (N=20,070) yields genetic overlap with schizophrenia and sex differences in heritability. Mol Psychiatry 23(3):666–673, 2018

Dunn J, Plomin R: Separate Lives: Why Siblings Are So Different. New York, Basic Books, 1990

Egeland JA, Hostetter AM: Amish Study, I: affective disorders among the Amish, 1976–1980. Am J Psychiatry 140(1):56–61, 1983

Eisenberg L: Mindlessness and brainlessness in psychiatry. Br J Psychiatry 148:497–508, 1986

Eisenberg L: The social construction of the human brain. Am J Psychiatry 152(11):1563–1575, 1995

Elkin I, Shea MT, Watkins JT, et al: National Institute of Mental Health Treatment of Depression Collaborative Research Program: general effectiveness of treatments. Arch Gen Psychiatry 46(11):971–982, 1989

Ellenberger HF: The Discovery of the Unconscious: The History and Evolution of Dynamic Psychiatry. New York, Basic Books, 1970

Elliott J, Shepherd P: Cohort profile: 1970 British Birth Cohort (BCS70). Int J Epidemiol 35(4):836–843, 2006

Elliott ML, Romer A, Knodt AR, Hariri AR: A connectome-wide functional signature of transdiagnostic risk for mental illness. Biol Psychiatry 84(6):452–459, 2018

Engel GL: The clinical application of the biopsychosocial model. Am J Psychiatry 137(5):535–544, 1980

Erlenmeyer-Kimling L, Squires-Wheeler E, Adamo UH, et al: The New York High-Risk Project: psychoses and Cluster A personality disorders in offspring of schizophrenic parents at 23 years of follow-up. Arch Gen Psychiatry 52(10):857–865, 1995

Falconer DS, Mackay TFC: Introduction to Quantitative Genetics, 4th Edition. New York, Pearson Prentice Hall, 1996

Falloon IRH, Boyd JL, McGill CW: Family Care of Schizophrenia: A Problem-Solving Approach to the Treatment of Mental Illness. New York, Guilford, 1984

Faraone SV, Larsson H: Genetics of attention deficit hyperactivity disorder. Mol Psychiatry 24(4):562–575, 2019

Faraone SV, Sergeant J, Gillberg C, Biederman J: The worldwide prevalence of ADHD: is it an American condition? World Psychiatry 2(2):104–113, 2003

Fava M, Alpert JE, Borus JS, et al: Patterns of personality disorder comorbidity in early-onset versus late-onset major depression. Am J Psychiatry 153(10):1308–1312, 1996

Faravelli C, Pallanti S: Recent life events and panic disorder. Am J Psychiatry 146(5):622–626, 1989

Feder A, Nestler EJ, Charney DS: Psychobiology and molecular genetics of resilience. Nat Rev Neurosci 10(6):446–457, 2009

Fergusson DM, Lynskey MT, Horwood J: Childhood sexual abuse and psychiatric disorder in young adulthood: I: prevalence of sexual abuse and factors associated with sexual abuse. J Am Acad Child Adolesc Psychiatry 35(10):1355–1364, 1996a

Fergusson DM, Horwood LJ, Lynskey MT: Childhood sexual abuse and psychiatric disorder in young adulthood: II: psychiatric outcomes of childhood sexual abuse. J Am Acad Child Adolesc Psychiatry 35(10):1365–1374, 1996b

Fergusson DM, Boden JM, Horwood LJ, et al: MAOA, abuse exposure and antisocial behaviour: 30-year longitudinal study. Br J Psychiatry 198(6):457–463, 2011a

Fergusson DM, Horwood LJ, Miller AL, Kennedy MA: Life stress, 5-HTTLPR and mental disorder: findings from a 30-year longitudinal study. Br J Psychiatry 198(2):129–135, 2011b

Ferrari AJ, Charlson FJ, Norman RE, et al: Burden of depressive disorders by country, sex, age, and year: findings from the Global Burden of Disease Study 2010. PLoS Med 10(11):e1001547, 2013

Finkelhor D, Hotaling G, Lewis IA, Smith C: Sexual abuse in a national survey of adult men and women: prevalence, characteristics, and risk factors. Child Abuse Negl 14(1):19–28, 1990

Fossati A, Madeddu F, Maffei C: Borderline personality disorder and childhood sexual abuse: a metanalytic study. J Pers Disord 13(3):268–280, 1999

Frances A: Saving Normal: An Insider's Revolt Against Out-of-Control Psychiatric Diagnosis, DSM-5, Big Pharma, and the Medicalization of Ordinary Life. New York, William Morrow, 2013

Frances A, Carroll B: Keith Conners (obituary). BMJ 358:j2253, 2017

Frank JD, Frank JB: Persuasion and Healing: A Comparative Study of Psychotherapy, 3rd Edition. Baltimore, MD, Johns Hopkins University Press, 1991

Friborg O, Martinsen EW, Martinussen M, et al: Comorbidity of personality disorders in mood disorders: a meta-analytic review of 122 studies from 1988 to 2010. J Affect Disord 152–154:1–11, 2014

Gabbard GO, Goodwin FK: Clinical psychiatry in transition: integrating biological and psychological perspectives, in Review of Psychiatry, Vol 15. Edited by Dickstein LJ, Riba MB, Oldham JM. Washington DC, American Psychiatric Press, 1996, pp 527–548

Garner DM, Garfinkel PE (eds): Handbook of Psychotherapy for Anorexia Nervosa and Bulimia. New York, Guilford, 1985

Geller DA: Obsessive-compulsive and spectrum disorders in children and adolescents. Psychiatr Clin North Am 29(2):353–370, 2006

Gellner E: The Psychoanalytic Movement: The Cunning of Unreason, Second Edition. London, Fontana, 1993

Geschwind DH, Flint J: Genetics and genomics of psychiatric disease. Science 349(6255):1489–1494, 2015

Gillett C: Reduction and Emergence in Science and Philosophy. Cambridge, UK, Cambridge University Press, 2016

Godfrey-Smith P: Philosophy of Biology (Princeton Foundations of Contemporary Philosophy). Princeton, NJ, Princeton University Press, 2014

Gold I: Reduction in psychiatry. Can J Psychiatry 54(8):506–512, 2009

Goldapple K, Segal Z, Garson C, et al: Modulation of cortical-limbic pathways in major depression: treatment-specific effects of cognitive behavior therapy. Arch Gen Psychiatry 61(1):34–41, 2004

Golding J: European Longitudinal Study of Pregnancy and Childhood (ELSPAC). Paediatric and Perinatal Epidemiology 3(4):460–469, 1989

Golding J, ALSPAC Study Team: The Avon Longitudinal Study of Parents and Children (ALSPAC)—study design and collaborative opportunities. Eur J Endocrinol 151 (suppl 3): U119–U123, 2004

Goldstein S, Brooks RB (eds): Handbook of Resilience in Children, 2nd Edition. New York, Springer, 2013

Goodwin DW, Warnock JK: Alcoholism: a family disease, in Clinical Textbook of Addictive Disorders. Edited by Frances RJ, Miller SI. New York, Guilford, 1991, pp 485–500

Gorman JM: Neuroscience at the Intersection of Mind and Brain. New York, Oxford University Press, 2018

Gottesman II: Schizophrenia Genesis: The Origins of Madness. New York, Freeman, 1991

Gottschalk MG, Domschke K: Genetics of generalized anxiety disorder and related traits. Dialogues Clin Neurosci 19(2):159–168, 2017

Gould TD, Gottesman II: Psychiatric endophenotypes and the development of valid animal models. Genes Brain Behav 5(2):113–119, 2006

Grant BF, Goldstein RB, Saha TD, et al: Epidemiology of DSM-5 alcohol use disorder: results from the National Epidemiologic Survey on Alcohol and Related Conditions III. JAMA Psychiatry 72(8):757–766, 2015

Grinker RR: Psychiatry rushes madly in all directions. Arch Gen Psychiatry 10:228–237, 1964

Grizenko N, Fortier ME, Zadorozny C, et al: Maternal stress during pregnancy, ADHD symptomatology in children and genotype: gene-environment interaction. J Can Acad Child Adolesc Psychiatry 21(1):9–15, 2012

Groenman AP, Janssen TWP, Oosterlaan J: Childhood psychiatric disorders as risk factor for subsequent substance abuse: a meta-analysis. J Am Acad Child Adolesc Psychiatry 56(7):556–569, 2017

Gross LS, Li L, Ford ES, Liu S: Increased consumption of refined carbohydrates and the epidemic of type 2 diabetes in the United States: an ecologic assessment. Am J Clin Nutr 79(5):774–779, 2004

Gull W: Proceedings of the Clinical Society of London. Br Med J 1:527–529, 1873

Guloksuz S, Pries L, Delespaul P: Examining the independent and joint effects of molecular genetic liability and environmental exposures in schizophrenia: results from the EUGEI study. World Psychiatry 18(2):173–182, 2019

Hale NG Jr: The Rise and Crisis of Psychoanalysis in the United States: Freud and the Americans, 1917–1985. New York, Oxford University Press, 1995

Hammen CL, Burge D, Daley SE, et al: Interpersonal attachment cognitions and prediction of symptomatic responses to interpersonal stress. J Abnorm Psychol 104(3):436–443, 1995

Hamshere ML, Stergiakouli E, Langley K, et al: Shared polygenic contribution between childhood attention-deficit hyperactivity disorder and adult schizophrenia. Br J Psychiatry 203(2):107–111, 2013

Hannon E, Knox O, Sugden K, et al: Characterizing genetic and environmental influences on variable DNA methylation using monozygotic and dizygotic twins. PLoS Genet 14(8):e1007544, 2018

Harding CM, Brooks GW, Ashikaga T, et al: The Vermont Longitudinal Study of persons with severe mental illness, II: long-term outcome of subjects who retrospectively met DSM-III criteria for schizophrenia. Am J Psychiatry 144(6):727–735, 1987

Harrington A: Mind Fixers: Psychiatry's Troubled Search for the Biology of Mental Illness. New York, WW Norton, 2019

Harris JR: The Nurture Assumption: Why Children Turn Out the Way They Do, 2nd Edition. New York, Free Press, 2009

Hechtman L (ed): Attention Deficit Hyperactivity Disorder: Adult Outcome and Its Predictors. New York, Oxford University Press, 2016

Heijmans BT, Tobi EW, Stein AD, et al: Persistent epigenetic differences associated with prenatal exposure to famine in humans. Proc Natl Acad Sci USA 105(44):17046–17049, 2008

Helzer JE, Canino GJ (eds): Alcoholism in North America, Europe, and Asia. New York, Oxford University Press, 1992

Hetherington EM: An overview of the Virginia Longitudinal Study of Divorce and Remarriage with a focus on early adolescence. Journal of Family Psychology 7(1):39–56, 1993

Hoek HW, Brown AS, Susser E: The Dutch Famine and schizophrenia spectrum disorders. Soc Psychiatry Psychiatr Epidemiol 33(8):373–379, 1998

Hollingshead AB, Redlich FC: Social Class and Mental Illness: Community Study. New York, Wiley, 1958

Hooley JM: Expressed emotion and relapse of psychopathology. Annu Rev Clin Psychol 3:329–352, 2007

Hopwood CJ, Mulay AL, Waugh MH (eds): The DSM-5 Alternative Model for Personality Disorders. New York, Routledge, 2019

Horwitz AV: PTSD: A Short History. Baltimore, MD, Johns Hopkins University Press, 2018

Horwitz AV, Wakefield JC: The Loss of Sadness: How Psychiatry Transformed Normal Sorrow Into Depressive Disorder. New York, Oxford University Press, 2007

Howard KI, Kopta SM, Krause MS, Orlinsky DE: The dose-effect relationship in psychotherapy. Am Psychol 41(2):159–164, 1986

Hübel C, Gaspar HA, Coleman JRI, et al: Genetic correlations of psychiatric traits with body composition and glycemic traits are sex- and age-dependent. Nat Commun 10(1):5765, 2019

Hunsley J, Elliott K, Therrien Z: The efficacy and effectiveness of psychological treatments for mood, anxiety, and related disorders. Can Psychol 55(3):161–176, 2014

Hwu HG, Yeh EK, Chang LY: Prevalence of psychiatric disorders in Taiwan defined by the Chinese Diagnostic Interview Schedule. Acta Psychiatr Scand 79(2):136–147, 1989

Hyman SE: The diagnosis of mental disorders: the problem of reification. Annu Rev Clin Psychol 6:155–179, 2010

Insel TR, Quirion R: Psychiatry as a clinical neuroscience discipline. JAMA 294(17):2221–2224, 2005

International Obsessive Compulsive Disorder Foundation Genetics Collaborative (IOCDF-GC) and OCD Collaborative Genetics Association Studies (OCGAS): Revealing the complex genetic architecture of obsessive-compulsive disorder using meta-analysis. Mol Psychiatry 23(5):1181–1188, 2018

Insel TR: The NIMH Research Domain Criteria (RDoC) Project: precision medicine for psychiatry. Am J Psychiatry 171(4):395–397, 2014

Ioannidis JPA: Contradicted and initially stronger effects in highly cited clinical research. JAMA 294(2):218–228, 2005

Jablensky A, Sartorius N, Ernberg G, et al: Schizophrenia: manifestations, incidence and course in different cultures. A World Health Organization ten-country study. Psychol Med Monogr Suppl 20:1–97, 1992

Jaffee SR: Child maltreatment and risk for psychopathology in childhood and adulthood. Annu Rev Clin Psychol 13:525–551, 2017

Jang KL, Livesley WJ, Vernon PA, Jackson DN: Heritability of personality disorder traits: a twin study. Acta Psychiatr Scand 94(6):438–444, 1996

Jellinek EM: The Disease Concept of Alcoholism. New Haven, CT, Hillhouse Press, 1960

Jensen KP: A review of genome-wide association studies of stimulant and opioid use disorders. Mol Neuropsychiatry 2(1):37–45, 2016

Jensen PS, Hoagwood K: The book of names: DSM–IV in context. Dev Psychopathol 9(2):231–249, 1997

Johnson EC, Border R, Melroy-Greif WE, et al: No evidence that schizophrenia candidate genes are more associated with schizophrenia than noncandidate genes. Biol Psychiatry 82(10):702–708, 2017

Kagan J: Galen's Prophecy: Temperament in Human Nature. New York, Basic Books, 1994

Kalin NH: Gaining ground on schizophrenia: conceptualizing how to use neuroimaging and genomics in its diagnosis and treatment. Am J Psychiatry 176(10):771–773, 2019

Kandel ER: The Disordered Mind: What Unusual Brains Tell Us About Ourselves. New York, Farrar, Straus & Giroux, 2018

Kanner L: Autistic disturbances of affective contact. Nervous Child 2:217–250, 1943

Kendler KS: Genetic epidemiology in psychiatry: taking both genes and environment seriously. Arch Gen Psychiatry 52(11):895–899, 1995

Kendler KS: From many to one to many—the search for causes of psychiatric illness. JAMA Psychiatry 76(10):1085–1091, 2019

Kendler KS, Eaves LJ: Models for the joint effect of genotype and environment on liability to psychiatric illness. Am J Psychiatry 143(3):279–289, 1986

Kendler KS, Prescott CA: Genes, Environment, and Psychopathology: Understanding the Causes of Psychiatric and Substance Use Disorders. New York, Guilford, 2006

Kendler KS, Heath AC, Martin NG, Eaves LJ: Symptoms of anxiety and symptoms of depression: same genes, different environments? Arch Gen Psychiatry 44(5):451–457, 1987

Kendler KS, MacLean C, Neale M, et al: The genetic epidemiology of bulimia nervosa. Am J Psychiatry 148(12):1627–1637, 1991a

Kendler KS, Kessler RC, Heath AC, et al: Coping: a genetic epidemiological investigation. Psychol Med 21(2):337–346, 1991b

Kendler KS, Neale MC, Kessler RC, et al: Familial influences on the clinical characteristics of major depression: a twin study. Acta Psychiatr Scand 86(5):371–378, 1992a

Kendler KS, Neale MC, Kessler RC, et al: Generalized anxiety disorder in women: a population-based twin study. Arch Gen Psychiatry 49(4):267–272, 1992b

Kendler KS, McGuire M, Gruenberg AM, et al: The Roscommon Family Study, I: methods, diagnosis of probands, and risk of schizophrenia in relatives. Arch Gen Psychiatry 50(7):527–540, 1993a

Kendler KS, Neale MC, Kessler RC, et al: A longitudinal twin study of personality and major depression in women. Arch Gen Psychiatry 50(11):853–862, 1993b

Kendler KS, Neale MC, Kessler RC, et al: Panic disorder in women: a population-based twin study. Psychol Med 23(2):397–406, 1993c

Kendler KS, Eaves LJ, Walters EE, et al: The identification and validation of distinct depressive syndromes in a population-based sample of female twins. Arch Gen Psychiatry 53(5):391–399, 1996

Kendler KS, Jacobson KC, Prescott CA, Neale MC: Specificity of genetic and environmental risk factors for use and abuse/dependence of cannabis, cocaine, hallucinogens, sedatives, stimulants, and opiates in male twins. Am J Psychiatry 160(4):687–695, 2003

Kendler KS, Kuhn JW, Prescott CA: Childhood sexual abuse, stressful life events and risk for major depression in women. Psychol Med 34(8):1475–1482, 2004

Kendler KS, Gatz M, Gardner CO, Pedersen NL: Personality and major depression: a Swedish longitudinal, population-based twin study. Arch Gen Psychiatry 63(10):1113–1120, 2006

Kendler KS, Gardner CO, Gatz M, Pedersen NL: The sources of co-morbidity between major depression and generalized anxiety disorder in a Swedish national twin sample. Psychol Med 37(3):453–462, 2007

Kendler KS, Larsson Lönn S, Salvatore J, et al: Divorce and the onset of alcohol use disorder: a Swedish population-based longitudinal cohort and co-relative study. Am J Psychiatry 174(5):451–458, 2017

Kendler KS, Ohlsson H, Lichtenstein P, et al: The genetic epidemiology of treated major depression in Sweden. Am J Psychiatry 175(11):1137–1144, 2018

Kendler KS, Aggen SH, Gillespie N, et al: The structure of genetic and environmental influences on normative personality, abnormal personality traits, and personality disorder symptoms. Psychol Med 49(8):1392–1399, 2019

Kessler RC, McGonagle KA, Swartz M, et al: Sex and depression in the National Comorbidity Survey. I: lifetime prevalence, chronicity and recurrence. J Affect Disord 29(2–3):85–96, 1993

Kessler RC, McGonagle KA, Zhao S, et al: Lifetime and 12-month prevalence of DSM-III-R psychiatric disorders in the United States: Results from the National Comorbidity Survey. Arch Gen Psychiatry 51(1):8–19, 1994

Kessler RC, Berglund P, Demler O, et al: Lifetime prevalence and age-of-onset distributions of DSM-IV disorders in the National Comorbidity Survey Replication. Arch Gen Psychiatry 62(6):593–602, 2005

Kieseppä T, Partonen T, Haukka J, et al: High concordance of bipolar I disorder in a nationwide sample of twins. Am J Psychiatry 161(10):1814–1821, 2004

Kirmayer LJ: Beyond the "new cross-cultural psychiatry": cultural biology, discursive psychology and the ironies of globalization. Transcult Psychiatry 43(1):126–144, 2006

Kirsch I: Review: benefits of antidepressants over placebo limited except in very severe depression. Evid Based Ment Health 13(2):49, 2010

Kirsch I, Deacon BJ, Huedo-Medina TB, et al: Initial severity and antidepressant benefits: a meta-analysis of data submitted to the Food and Drug Administration. PLoS Med 5(2):e45, 2008

Klerman G: Historical perspectives on contemporary schools of psychopathology, in Contemporary Directions in Psychopathology: Toward the DSM-IV. Edited by Millon T, Klerman G. New York, Guilford, 1986, pp 3–28

Klerman GL, Weissman MM: Increasing rates of depression. JAMA 261(15):2229–2235, 1989

Knopik V, Neiderhiser JM, DeFries JC, Plomin R: Behavioral Genetics, 7th Edition. New York, WH Freeman, 2017

Knudson AG: Hereditary cancer: two hits revisited. J Cancer Res Clin Oncol 122(3):135–140, 1996

Kocsis JH, Sutton BM, Frances AJ: Long-term follow-up of chronic depression treated with imipramine. J Clin Psychiatry 52(2):56–59, 1991

Kotov R, Perlman G, GámezW, Watson D: The structure and short-term stability of the emotional disorders: a dimensional approach. Psychol Med 45(8):1687–1698, 2015

Kotov R, Krueger RF, Watson D, et al: The Hierarchical Taxonomy of Psychopathology (HiTOP): a dimensional alternative to traditional nosologies. J Abnorm Psychol 126(4):454–477, 2017

Kraemer HC, Kazdin AE, Offord DR, et al: Coming to terms with the terms of risk. Arch Gen Psychiatry 54(4):337–343, 1997

Kraepelin E: Dementia Praecox and Paraphrenia. Translated by Barclay RM and edited by Robertson GM. Edinburgh, E & S Livingstone, 1919

Krueger RF, Johnson W: The Minnesota Twin Registry: current status and future directions. Twin Res 5(5):488–492, 2002

Krueger RF, Markon KE: Reinterpreting comorbidity: a model-based approach to understanding and classifying psychopathology. Annu Rev Clin Psychol 2:111–133, 2006

Krueger RF, Tackett JL: Personality and psychopathology: working toward the bigger picture. J Pers Disord 17(2):101–128, 2003

Kumsta R, Stevens S, Brookes K, et al: 5HTT genotype moderates the influence of early institutional deprivation on emotional problems in adolescence: evidence from the English and Romanian Adoptee (ERA) Study. J Child Psychol Psychiatry 51(7):755–762, 2010

Kupfer DJ, Regier DA: Neuroscience, clinical evidence, and the future of psychiatric classification in DSM-5. Am J Psychiatry 168(7):672–674, 2011

Lambert MJ (ed): Bergin and Garfield's Handbook of Psychotherapy and Behavior Change, 6th Edition. New York, Wiley, 2013

Landberg J, Danielsson A-K, Falkstedt D, Hemmingsson T: Fathers' alcohol consumption and long-term risk for mortality in offspring. Alcohol Alcohol 53(6):753–759, 2018

Laporte L, Paris J, Guttman H, Russell J: Psychopathology, childhood trauma, and personality traits in patients with borderline personality disorder and their sisters. J Pers Disord 25(4):448–462, 2011

Laufer RS, Gallops MS, Frey-Wouters E: War stress and trauma: the Vietnam veteran experience. J Health Soc Behav 25(1):65–85, 1984

Lee KA, Vaillant GE, Torrey WC, Elder GH: A 50-year prospective study of the psychological sequelae of World War II combat. Am J Psychiatry 152(4):516–522, 1995

Leff JP: Psychiatry Around the Globe: A Transcultural View (Gaskell Psychiatry Series). London, Gaskell, 1988

Leighton DC, Harding JS, Macklin DB: The Character of Danger: Psychiatric Symptoms in Selected Communities. New York, Basic Books, 1963

Lenzenweger MF: Epidemiology of personality disorders. Psychiatr Clin North Am 31(3):395–403, 2008

Leo J: Schizophrenia adoption studies. PLoS Med 3(8):e366, 2006

Leucht S, Hierl S, Kissling W, et al: Putting the efficacy of psychiatric and general medicine medication into perspective: review of meta-analyses. Br J Psychiatry 200(2):97–206, 2012

Levey DF, Gelernter J, Polimanti R, et al: Reproducible genetic risk loci for anxiety: results from 200,000 participants in the Million Veteran Program. Am J Psychiatry 177(3):223–232, 2020

Levy DL, Mendell NR, Holzman PS: The antisaccade task and neuropsychological tests of prefrontal cortical integrity in schizophrenia: empirical findings and interpretative considerations. World Psychiatry 3(1):32–40, 2004

Lewinsohn PM, Mischel W, Chaplin W, Barton R: Social competence and depression: the role of illusory self-perceptions. J Abnorm Psychol 89(2):203–212, 1980

Lewis L, Appleby L: Personality disorder: the patients psychiatrists dislike. Br J Psychiatry 153:44–49, 1988

Lewontin RC, Rose S, Kamin LJ: Not in Our Genes: Biology, Ideology and Human Nature. London, Pantheon Books, 1984

Li D, Sham PC, Owen MJ, He L: Meta-analysis shows significant association between dopamine system genes and attention deficit hyperactivity disorder (ADHD). Hum Mol Genet 15(14):2276–2284, 2006

Li D, Chang X, Connolly JJ, et al: A genome-wide association study of anorexia nervosa suggests a risk locus implicated in dysregulated leptin signaling. Sci Rep 7(1):3847, 2017

Lichtenstein P, Yip BH, Björk C, et al: Common genetic determinants of schizophrenia and bipolar disorder in Swedish families: a population-based study. Lancet 373(9659):234–239, 2009

Linehan MM: Cognitive-Behavioral Treatment of Borderline Personality Disorder. New York, Guilford, 1993

Lipowski ZJ: Psychiatry: mindless or brainless, both or neither? Can J Psychiatry 34(3):249–254, 1989

Lippard ETC, Nemeroff CB: The devastating clinical consequences of child abuse and neglect: increased disease vulnerability and poor treatment response in mood disorders. Am J Psychiatry 177(1):20–36, 2020

Liu CC, Liu CC, Kanekiyo T, et al: Apolipoprotein E and Alzheimer disease: risk, mechanisms and therapy Nat Rev Neurol 9(2):106–118, 2013

Livesley WJ: Practical Management of Personality Disorder. New York, Guilford, 2003

Loftus EF: The reality of repressed memories. Am Psychol 48(5):518–537, 1993

Lvovs D, Favorova OO, Favorov AV: A polygenic approach to the study of polygenic diseases. Acta Naturae 4(3):59–71, 2012

Lyons MJ, Goldberg J, Eisen SA, et al: Do genes influence exposure to trauma? A twin study of combat. Am J Med Genet 48(1):22–27, 1993

Malinosky-Rummell R, Hansen DJ: Long-term consequences of childhood physical abuse. Psychol Bull 114(1):68–79, 1993

Manolio TA, Collins FS, Cox NJ, et al: Finding the missing heritability of complex diseases. Nature 461(7265):747–753, 2009

Marmot MG, Smith GD, Stansfeld S, et al: Health inequalities among British civil servants: the Whitehall II study. Lancet 337(8754):1387–1393, 1991

Masten AS, Cicchetti D: Developmental cascades. Dev Psychopathol 22(3):491–495, 2010

Mattheisen M, Samuels JF, Wang Y, et al: Genome-wide association study in obsessive-compulsive disorder: results from the OCGAS. Mol Psychiatry 20(3):337–344, 2015

May PRA: The Treatment of Schizophrenia. New York, Science House, 1968

Mayhew AJ, Pigeyre M, Couturier J, Meyre D: An evolutionary genetic perspective of eating disorders. Neuroendocrinology 106(3):292–306, 2018

Maynard TM, Sikich L, Lieberman JA, LaMantia AS: Neural development, cell-cell signaling, and the "two-hit" hypothesis of schizophrenia. Schizophr Bull 27(3):457–476, 2001

McFarlane AC: Vulnerability to posttraumatic stress disorder, in Posttraumatic Stress Disorder: Etiology, Phenomenology, and Treatment. Edited by Wolf ME, Mosnaim AD. Washington, DC, American Psychiatric Press, 1990, pp 3–20

McGuffin P, Gottesman I: Genetic influences on normal and abnormal development, in Child and Adolescent Psychiatry: Modern Approaches. Edited by Rutter M, Hersov L. Oxford, UK, Blackwell, 1985, pp 17–33

McGuffin P, Katz R, Rutherford J: Nature, nurture and depression: a twin study. Psychol Med 21(2):329–335, 1991

McGuffin P, Katz R, Watkins S, Rutherford J: A hospital-based twin register of the heritability of DSM-IV unipolar depression. Arch Gen Psychiatry 53(2):129–136, 1996

McGuffin P, Rijsjdijk F, Andrew MP, et al: The heritability of bipolar affective disorder and the genetic relationship to unipolar depression. Arch Gen Psychiatry 60(5):497–502, 2003

McGuffin P, Owen MJ, Gottesman I (eds): Psychiatric Genetics and Genomics. New York, Oxford University Press, 2004

McGuire M, Troisi A: Darwinian Psychiatry. New York: Oxford University Press, 1998

McLanahan S, Tach L, Schneider D: The causal effects of father absence. Annu Rev Sociol 39:399–427, 2013

McLaughlin KA, Hatzenbuehler ML: Stressful life events, anxiety sensitivity, and internalizing symptoms in adolescents. J Abnorm Psychol 118(3):659–669, 2009

McLaughlin KA, Conron KJ, Koenen KC, Gilman SE: Childhood adversity, adult stressful life events, and risk of past-year psychiatric disorder: a test of the stress sensitization hypothesis in a population-based sample of adults. Psychol Med 40(10):1647–1658, 2010a

McLaughlin KA, Kubzansky LD, Dunn EC, et al: Childhood social environment, emotional reactivity to stress, and mood and anxiety disorders across the life course. Depress Anxiety 27(12):1087–1094, 2010b

McNally RJ: Remembering Trauma. Cambridge, MA, Belknap Press, 2003

Meaney MJ, Ferguson-Smith NC: Epigenetic regulation of the neural transcriptome: the meaning of the marks. Nat Neurosci 13(11):1313–1318, 2010

Meehl PE: Toward an integrated theory of schizotaxa, schizotypy, and schizophrenia. J Pers Disord 4(1):1–99, 1990

Millan MJ, Andrieux A, Bartzokis G, et al: Altering the course of schizophrenia: progress and perspectives. Nat Rev Drug Discov 15(7):485–515, 2016

Millon T, Davis RD: Disorders of Personality: DSM-IV and Beyond, 2nd Edition. New York, Wiley, 1996

Mitchell MR, Potenza MN: Addictions and personality traits: impulsivity and related constructs. Curr Behav Neurosci Rep 1(1):1–12, 2014

Moffitt TE, Caspi A, Rutter MM, Silva PA: Sex Differences in Antisocial Behaviour: Conduct Disorder, Delinquency, and Violence in the Dunedin Longitudinal Study. Cambridge, UK, Cambridge University Press, 2001

Moffitt TE, Houts R, Asherson P, et al: Is adult ADHD a childhood-onset neurodevelopmental disorder? Evidence from a four-decade longitudinal cohort study. Am J Psychiatry 172(10):967–977, 2015

Moncrieff J: A critique of the dopamine hypothesis of schizophrenia and psychosis. Harv Rev Psychiatry 17(3):214–225, 2009

Moncrieff J: Research on a "drug-centred" approach to psychiatric drug treatment: assessing the impact of mental and behavioural alterations produced by psychiatric drugs. Epidemiol Psychiatr Sci 27(2):133–140, 2018

Mojtabai R: Increase in antidepressant medication in the US adult population between 1990 and 2003. Psychother Psychosom 77(2):83–92, 2008

Monroe SM, Simons AD: Diathesis-stress theories in the context of life stress research: implications for the depressive disorders. Psychol Bull 110(3):406–425, 1991

Moreira PS, Marques P, Soriano-Mas C, et al: The neural correlates of obsessive-compulsive disorder: a multimodal perspective. Transl Psychiatry 7(8):e1224, 2017

Morgan C, Charalambides M, Hutchinson G, Murray RM: Migration, ethnicity, and psychosis: toward a sociodevelopmental model. Schizophr Bull 36(4):655–664, 2010

Morgan C, Gayer-Anderson C: Childhood adversities and psychosis: evidence, challenges, implications. World Psychiatry 15(2):93–102, 2016

Morgan C, Knowles G, Hutchinson G: Migration, ethnicity and psychoses: evidence, models and future direction. World Psychiatry 18(3):247–258, 2019

Mosing MA, Gordon SD, Medland SE, et al: Genetic and environmental influences on the co-morbidity between depression, panic disorder, agoraphobia, and social phobia: a twin study. Depress Anxiety 26(11):1004–1011, 2009

Muncie W: Psychobiology and Psychiatry. St Louis, MO, CV Mosby, 1939

Murphy HBM: Comparative Psychiatry: The International and Intercultural Distribution of Mental Illness. New York, Springer, 1982

National Institute for Health and Care Excellence: Personality disorders: borderline and antisocial (Quality Standard [QS88]. [London], National Institute for Health and Care Excellence, 2015. Available at: https://www.nice.org.uk/guidance/qs88. Accessed February 14, 2020.

Nesse RM: Good Reasons for Bad Feelings: Insights From the Frontier of Evolutionary Psychiatry. New York, Dutton, 2019

Nesse RM, Williams GC: Evolution and Healing: The New Science of Darwinian Medicine, 2nd Edition. London, Orion Publishing, 1995

Nesse RM, Williams GC: Why We Get Sick: The New Science of Darwinian Medicine. New York, Random House, 1994

Newton-Howes G, Tyrer P, Johnson T: Personality disorder and the outcome of depression: meta-analysis of published studies. Br J Psychiatry 188:13–20, 2006

Nock MK, Kazdin AE, Hiripi E, Kessler RC: Prevalence, subtypes, and correlates of DSM-IV conduct disorder in the National Comorbidity Survey Replication. Psychol Med 36(5):699–710, 2006

Nurnberger JL, Gershon ES: Genetics, in Handbook of Affective Disorders, 2nd Edition. Edited by Paykel ES. New York, Guilford, 1992, pp 131–148

Oetting ER, Donnermeyer JF, Trimble JE, Beauvais F: Primary socialization theory: culture, ethnicity, and cultural identification. The links between culture and substance use, IV. Subst Use Misuse 33(10):2075–2107, 1998

Olfson M, Marcus SC: National trends in outpatient psychotherapy. Am J Psychiatry 167(12):1456–1463, 2010

Olfson M, Blanco C, Wang S, Greenhill LL: Trends in office-based treatment of adults with stimulants in the United States. J Clin Psychiatry 74(1):43–50, 2013

Ong AD, Bergeman CS, Boker SM: Resilience comes of age: defining features in later adulthood. J Pers 77(6):1777–1804, 2009

Ostergaard SD, Larsen JT, Dalsgaard S, et al: Predicting ADHD by assessment of Rutter's indicators of adversity in infancy. PloS One 11(6):0157352, 2016

Pan LA, Goldstein TR, Rooks BT, et al: The relationship between stressful life events and Axis I diagnoses among adolescent offspring of probands with bipolar and non-bipolar psychiatric disorders and healthy controls: the Pittsburgh Bipolar Offspring Study (BIOS). J Clin Psychiatry 78(3):e234–e243, 2017

Paris J: Social Factors in the Personality Disorders: A Biopsychosocial Approach to Etiology and Treatment. Cambridge, UK, Cambridge University Press, 1996

Paris J: The Use and Misuse of Psychiatric Drugs: An Evidence-Based Guide. London, Wiley, 2010

Paris J: The Bipolar Spectrum: Diagnosis or Fad? New York, Routledge, 2012

Paris J: The Intelligent Clinician's Guide to DSM-5, 2nd Edition. New York, Oxford University Press, 2015a

Paris J: Overdiagnosis in Psychiatry: How Modern Psychiatry Lost Its Way While Creating a Diagnosis for Almost All of Life's Misfortunes. New York, Oxford University Press, 2015b

Paris J: Stepped Care for Borderline Personality Disorder: Making Treatment Brief, Effective, and Accessible. New York, Academic Press, 2017

Paris J: An Evidence-Based Critique of Contemporary Psychoanalysis: Research, Theory, and Clinical Practice. London, Routledge, 2019

Paris J: Treatment of Borderline Personality Disorder: A Guide to Evidence-Based Practice, 2nd Edition. New York, Guilford, 2020

Paris J, Kirmayer LJ: The National Institute of Mental Health Research Domain Criteria: a bridge too far. J Nerv Ment Dis 204(1):26–32, 2016

Paris J, Zweig-Frank H, Guzder J: Psychological risk factors for borderline personality disorder in female patients. Compr Psychiatry 35:301–305, 1994

Paris J, Bhat V, Thombs B: Is adult attention-deficit hyperactivity disorder being overdiagnosed? Can J Psychiatry 60(7):324–328, 2015

Parker G: Parental Overprotection: A Risk Factor in Psychosocial Development. New York, Grune & Stratton, 1983

Parker G, Bassett D, Outhred T, et al: Defining melancholia: a core mood disorder. Bipolar Disord 19(3):235–237, 2017

Parnas J: Psychiatry without the Psyche. World Psychiatry 13:46–47, 2014

Parrington J: The Deeper Genome: Why There Is More to the Human Genome Than Meets the Eye. New York, Oxford University Press, 2015

Paykel ES (ed): Handbook of Affective Disorders, 2nd Edition. New York, Churchill Livingstone, 1992

Paykel ES: Life events and affective disorders. Acta Psychiat Scand Suppl 108 (suppl 418):61–66, 2003

Pepper CM, Klein DN, Anderson RL, et al: DSM-III-R Axis II comorbidity in dysthymia and major depression. Am J Psychiatry 152(2):239–247, 1995

Peterson CB, Thuras P, Ackard DM, et al: Personality dimensions in bulimia nervosa, binge eating disorder, and obesity. Compr Psychiatry 51(1):31–36, 2010

Peyrot WJ, Van der Auwera S, Milaneschi Y, et al: Does childhood trauma moderate polygenic risk for depression? A meta-analysis of 5765 subjects from the Psychiatric Genomics Consortium. Biol Psychiatry 84(2):138–147, 2018

Pike A, McGuire S, Hetherington EM, et al: Family environment and adolescent depressive symptoms and antisocial behavior: a multivariate genetic analysis. Developmental Psychol 32(4):590–603, 1996

Pinker S: The Blank Slate: The Modern Denial of Human Nature. New York, Viking, 2002

Pinker S: The Language Instinct: How the Mind Creates Language. New York, Harper Perennial Modern Classics, 2007

Pinker S: Enlightenment Now: The Case for Reason, Science, Humanism, and Progress. New York, Viking, 2018

Plomin R: The role of inheritance in behavior. Science 248(4952):183–188, 1990

Plomin R: The Emanuel Miller Memorial Lecture 1993: genetic research and identification of environmental influences. J Child Psychol Psychiatry 35(5):817–834, 1994

Plomin R: Blueprint: How DNA Makes Us Who We Are. Cambridge, MA, MIT Press, 2018

Plomin R, DeFries JC, Knopik VS, Neiderhiser JN: Behavioral Genetics, 6th Edition. New York, MacMillan, 2013

Plomin R, DeFries JC, Knopik VS, Neiderhiser JM: Top 10 replicated findings from behavioral genetics. Perspect Psychol Sci 11(1):3–23, 2016

Polderman TJC, Benyamin B, de Leeuw CA, et al: Meta-analysis of the heritability of human traits based on fifty years of twin studies. Nat Genet 47(7):702–709, 2015

Post RM: Transduction of psychosocial stress into the neurobiology of recurrent affective disorder. Am J Psychiatry 149(8):999–1010, 1992

Poulton R, Moffitt TE, Silva PA: The Dunedin Multidisciplinary Health and Development Study: overview of the first 40 years, with an eye to the future. Soc Psychiatry Psychiatr Epidemiol 50(5): 679–693, 2015

Power C, Elliott J: Cohort profile: 1958 British birth cohort (National Child Development Study). Int J Epidemiol 35(1):34–41, 2006

Power RA, Tansey KE, Buttenschøn HN, et al: Genome-wide association for major depression through age at onset stratification: Major Depressive Disorder Working Group of the Psychiatric Genomics Consortium. Biol Psychiatry 81(4):325–335, 2017

Poznik GD, Adamska K, Xu X, et al: A novel framework for sib pair linkage analysis. Am J Hum Genet 78(2):222–230, 2006

Pratt LA, Brody DJ, Gu Q: Antidepressant Use Among Persons Aged 12 and Over: United States, 2011–2014 (NCHS Data Brief No. 283). Washington, DC, National Center for Health Statistics, 2017

Prince R, Tcheng-Laroche F: Culture-bound syndromes and international disease classification. Cult Med Psychiatry 11(1):3–52, 1987

Rahe RH: Stress and psychiatry, in Comprehensive Textbook of Psychiatry, 6th Edition. Edited by Kaplan HI, Sadock BJ. Baltimore, MD, Williams & Wilkins, 1995, pp 1545–1559

Rasic D, Hajek T, Alda M, Uher R: Risk of mental illness in offspring of parents with schizophrenia, bipolar disorder, and major depressive disorder: a meta-analysis of family high-risk studies. Schizophr Bull 40(1):28–38, 2014

Råstam M, Gillberg G: The family background in anorexia nervosa: a population-based study. J Amer Acad Child Adolesc Psychiatry 30(2):283–289, 1991

Regier DA, Burke JD: Epidemiology, in Comprehensive Textbook of Psychiatry, 6th Edition. Edited by Kaplan HI, Sadock BJ. Baltimore, MD, Williams & Wilkins, 1995, pp 377–396

Regier DA, Narrow WE, Clarke DE, et al: DSM-5 field trials in the United States and Canada, Part II: test-retest reliability of selected categorical diagnoses. Am J Psychiatry 170(1):59–70, 2013

Reichborn-Kjennerud T, Ystrom E, Neale MC, et al: Structure of genetic and environmental risk factors for symptoms of DSM-IV borderline personality disorder. JAMA Psychiatry 70(11):1206–1214, 2013

Rhee SH, Waldman ID: Genetic and environmental influences on antisocial behavior: a meta-analysis of twin and adoption studies. Psychol Bull 128(3):490–529, 2002

Riglin L, Collishaw S, Richards A, et al: Schizophrenia risk alleles and neurodevelopmental outcomes in childhood: a population-based cohort study. Lancet Psychiatry 4(1):57–62, 2017

Rioux C, Castellanos-Ryan N, Parent S, et al. Age of cannabis use onset and adult drug abuse symptoms: a prospective study of common risk factors and indirect effects. Can J Psychiatry 63(7):457–464, 2018a

Rioux C, Séguin JR, Paris J: Differential susceptibility to the environment and borderline personality disorder. Harv Rev Psychiatry 26(6):374–383, 2018b

Riso LP, Klein DN, Ferro T, et al: Understanding the comorbidity between early-onset dysthymia and cluster B personality disorders: a family study. Am J Psychiatry 153(7):900–906, 1996

Robins E, Guze SB: Establishment of diagnostic validity in psychiatric illness: its application to schizophrenia. Am J Psychiatry 126(7):983–987, 1970

Robins LN: Deviant Children Grown-up: A Sociological and Psychiatric Study of Sociopathic Personality. Baltimore, MD, Williams & Wilkins, 1966

Robins LN, Regier DA (eds): Psychiatric Disorders in America: The Epidemiologic Catchment Area Study. New York, Free Press, 1991

Rosenbaum JF, Biederman J, Bolduc-Murphy EA, et al: Behavioral inhibition in childhood: a risk factor for anxiety disorders. Harv Rev Psychiatry 1(1):2–16, 1993

Rosenthal D: The Genain Quadruplets: A Case Study and Theoretical Analysis of Heredity and Environment in Schizophrenia. New York, Basic Books, 1963

Rosenvinge JH, Martinussen M, Ostensen E: The comorbidity of eating disorders and personality disorders: a meta-analytic review of studies published between 1983 and 1998. Eat Weight Disord 5(2):52–61, 2000

Rothbart MK, Ahadi SA, Evans DE: Temperament and personality: origins and outcomes. J Per Soc Psychol 78(1):122–135, 2000

Rowe DC: Environmental and genetic influences on dimensions of perceived parenting: a twin study. Dev Psychol 17(2):203–208, 1981

Rumyantsev SN: Observations on constitutional resistance to infection. Immunol Today 13(5):184–187, 1992

Rush AJ, Trivedi MH, Wisniewski SR, et al: Bupropion-SR, sertraline, or venlafaxine-XR after failure of SSRIs for depression. N Engl J Med 354(12):1231–1242, 2006

Rutter M: Psychosocial resilience and protective mechanisms. Am J Orthopsychiatry 57(3):316–331, 1987a

Rutter M: Temperament, personality and personality disorder. Br J Psychiatry 150:443–448, 1987b

Rutter M: Pathways from childhood to adult life. J Child Psychol Psychiatry 30(1):23–51, 1989

Rutter M: Genes and Behavior: Nature-Nurture Interplay Explained. Malden, MA, Blackwell, 2006

Rutter M: Resilience as a dynamic concept. Dev Psychopathol 24(2):335–344, 2012

Rutter M: Annual research review: resilience—clinical implications. J Child Psychol Psychiatry 54(4):474–487, 2013

Rutter M, Quinton D: Long-term follow-up of women institutionalized in childhood: factors promoting good functioning in adult life. Br J Dev Psychol 2(3):191–204, 1984

Rutter M, Smith D: Psychosocial Disorders in Young People: Time Trends and Their Causes. New York, Wiley, 1995

Rutter M, Cox A, Tupling C, et al: Attainment and adjustment in two geographical areas: I—the prevalence of psychiatric disorder. Br J Psychiatry 126:493–509, 1975

Rutter M, Moffitt TE, Caspi A: Gene-environment interplay and psychopathology: multiple varieties but real effects. J Child Psychol Psychiatry 47(3–4):226–261, 2006

Rutter M, Kumsta R, Schlotz W, Sonuga-Barke E: Longitudinal studies using a "natural experiment" design: the case of adoptees from Romanian institutions. J Am Acad Child Adoles Psychiatry 51(8):762–770, 2012

Salvatore JE, Dick DM: Genetic influences on conduct disorder. Neurosci Biobehav Rev 91:91–101, 2018

Scarr S: The construction of family reality. Behav Brain Sci 14:403–404, 1991

Scarr S, McCartney K: How people make their own environments: a theory of genotype greater than environment effects. Child Dev 54(2):424–435, 1983

Schuckit MA: Biological markers in alcoholism. Progr Neuropsychopharmacol Biol Psychiatry 10:191–199, 1986

Schuckit MA: A brief history of research on the genetics of alcohol and other drug use disorders. J Stud Alcohol Drugs Suppl 75 (suppl 17):59–67, 2014

Scourfield J, Van den Bree M, Martin N, McGuffin P: Conduct problems in children and adolescents: a twin study. Arch Gen Psychiatry 61(5):489–496, 2004

Seemüller F, Möller H-J, Dittman S, Musil R: Is the efficacy of psychopharmacological drugs comparable to the efficacy of general medicine medication? BMC Med 10: 17, 2012

Seeman P, Guan HC, Nobrega J, et al: Dopamine D2-like sites in schizophrenia, but not in Alzheimer's, Huntington's, or control brains, for [3H]benzquinoline. Synapse 25(2):137–146, 1997

Segerstråle U: Defenders of the Truth: The Sociobiology Debate. Oxford, UK, Oxford University Press, 2000

Shadrina M, Bondarenko EA, Slominsky PA: Genetic factors in major depression disease. Front Psychiatry 9:334, 2018

Sharon A, Levav I, Brodsky J, et al: Psychiatric disorders and other health dimensions among Holocaust survivors 6 decades later. Br J Psychiatry 195(4):331–335, 2009

Shea TM, Widiger TA, Klein MH: Comorbidity of personality disorders and depression implications for treatment. J Consult Clin Psychol 60:857–868, 1992

Shea MT, Elkin I, Imber SD, et al: Course of depressive symptoms over follow-up: Findings from the National Institute of Mental Health Treatment of Depression Collaborative Research Program. Arch Gen Psychiatry 49(10):782–787, 1992

Sheerin CM, Lind MJ, Bountress KE, et al: The genetics and epigenetics of PTSD: overview, recent advances, and future directions. Curr Opin Psychol 14:5–11, 2017

Sheerin CM, Lind MJ, Brown EA, et al: The impact of resilience and subsequent stressful life events on MDD and GAD. Depress Anxiety 35(2):140–147, 2018

Shiner RL: The development of personality disorders: perspectives from normal personality development in childhood and adolescence. Dev Psychopathol 21(3):715–734, 2009

Shorter E: A History of Psychiatry: From the Era of the Asylum to the Age of Prozac. New York, Wiley, 1997

Sideli L, Mulè A, La Barbera D, Murray RM: Do child abuse and maltreatment increase risk of schizophrenia? Psychiatry Investig 9(2):87–99, 2012

Sigvardsson S, Bohman M, Cloninger CR: Replication of the Stockholm Adoption Study of alcoholism: confirmatory cross-fostering analysis. Arch Gen Psychiatry 53(8):681–687, 1996

Slavich GM, Monroe SM, Gotlib IH: Early parental loss and depression history: associations with recent life stress in major depressive disorder. J Psychiatr Res 45(9):1146–1152, 2011

Smink FRE, van Hoeken D, Hoek HW: Epidemiology of eating disorders: incidence, prevalence and mortality rates. Curr Psychiatry Rep 14(4):406–414, 2012

Snow CP: The Two Cultures (1958). Cambridge, UK, Cambridge University Press, 1993

Sonuga-Barke EJ, Kennedy MK, Kumsta R, et al: Child-to-adult neurodevelopmental and mental health trajectories after early life deprivation: the young adult follow-up of the longitudinal English and Romanian adoptees study. Lancet 389(10078):1539–1548, 2017

Sørensen TI, Nielsen GG, Andersen PK, Teasdale TW: Genetic and environmental influences on premature death in adult adoptees. N Engl J Med 318(12):727–732, 1988

Southwick SM, Morgan CA III, Nicolaou AL, Charney DS: Consistency of memory for combat-related traumatic events in veterans of Operation Desert Storm. Am J Psychiatry 154(2):173–177, 1997

Sowell T: Intellectuals and Society. New York, Basic Books, 2010

Spanagel R: Animal models of addiction. Dialogues Clin Neurosci 19(3):247–258, 2017

Spencer TJ: ADHD and comorbidity in childhood. J Clin Psychiatry 67 (suppl 8):27–31, 2006

Srole L, Fischer AK: The Midtown Manhattan Longitudinal Study vs "the Mental Paradise Lost" doctrine. Arch Gen Psychiatry 37(2):209–221, 1980

Staley D, Wand RR: Obsessive-compulsive disorder: a review of the cross-cultural epidemiological literature. Transcultural Psychiatric Research Review 32(2):103–136, 1995

Steiger H, Richardson J, Joober R, et al: The 5HTTLPR polymorphism, prior maltreatment and dramatic-erratic personality manifestations in women with bulimic syndromes. J Psychiatry Neurosci 32(5):54–362, 2007

Stein MB, Jang KL, Taylor S, et al: Genetic and environmental influences on trauma exposure and posttraumatic stress disorder symptoms: a twin study. Am J Psychiatry 159(10):1675–1681, 2002

Stepp SD, Whalen DJ, Pilkonis PA, et al: Children of mothers with borderline personality disorder: identifying parenting behaviors as potential targets for intervention. Personal Disord 3(1):76–91, 2012

Stepp SD, Whalen DJ, Scott LN, et al: Reciprocal effects of parenting and borderline personality disorder symptoms in adolescent girls. Dev Psychopathol 26(2):361–378, 2014

Stepp SD, Scott LN, Jones NP, et al: Negative emotional reactivity as a marker of vulnerability in the development of borderline personality disorder symptoms. Dev Psychopathol 28(1):213–224, 2016

Stevens A, Price J: Evolutionary Psychiatry: A New Beginning, 2nd Edition. New York, Routledge, 2000

Still GF: The Goulstonian Lectures on some abnormal psychical conditions in children. Lancet 1:1008–1012, 1902

Stunkard AJ, Sørenson TI, Hanis C, et al: An adoption study of human obesity. N Engl J Med 314(4):193–198, 1986

Sullivan PF: The genetics of schizophrenia. PLoS Med 2(7):e212, 2005

Sullivan PF: The Psychiatric GWAS Consortium: big science comes to psychiatry. Neuron 68(2):182–186, 2010

Sullivan PF, Neale MC, Kendler KS: Genetic epidemiology of major depression: review and meta-analysis. Am J Psychiatry 157(10):1552–1562, 2000

Sullivan PF, Kendler KS, Neale MC: Schizophrenia as a complex trait: evidence from a meta-analysis of twin studies. Arch Gen Psychiatry 60(12):1187–1192, 2003

Tabery J: Beyond Versus: The Struggle to Understand the Interaction of Nature and Nurture. Cambridge, MA, MIT Press, 2014

Tang SX, Moore TM, Calkins ME, et al: Emergent, remitted and persistent psychosis-spectrum symptoms in 22q11.2 deletion syndrome. Transl Psychiatry 7(7):e1180, 2017

Tarter RE, Moss HB, Vanyukov MM: Behavioral genetics and the etiology of alcoholism, in The Genetics of Alcoholism. Edited by Begleiter H, Kissin B. New York, Oxford University Press, 1995, pp 294–326

Taylor S: Etiology of obsessions and compulsions: a meta-analysis and narrative review of twin studies. Clin Psychol Rev 31:1361–1372, 2011

TeareDM (ed): Genetic Epidemiology (Methods in Molecular Biology 713). New York, Humana, 2011

Tellegen A, Lykken DT, Bouchard TJ Jr, et al: Personality similarity in twins reared apart and together. J Pers Soc Psychol 54(6):1031–1039, 1988

Thapar A, Cooper M: Attention deficit hyperactivity disorder. Lancet 387(10024):1240–1250, 2016

Tong C, Wen L, Xia Y, et al: Protocol for a longitudinal twin birth cohort study to unravel the complex interplay between early life environmental and genetic risk factors in health and disease: the Chongqing Longitudinal Twin Study (LoTiS). BMJ Open 8(2):e017889, 2018

Torgersen S: Genetic factors in anxiety disorders. Arch Gen Psychiatry 40(10):1085–1089, 1983

Torgersen S, Myers J, Reichborn-Kjennerud T, et al: The heritability of Cluster B personality disorders assessed both by personal interview and questionnaire. J Pers Disord 26(6):848–866, 2012

Trace SE, Baker JH, Peñas-Lledó E, Bulik CM: The genetics of eating disorders Annu Rev Clin Psychol 9:589–620, 2013

Treasure J, Holland AJ: Genetic factors in eating disorders, in Handbook of Eating Disorders: Theory, Treatment and Research. Edited by Szmukler GI, Dare C, Treasure J. Chichester, UK, Wiley, 1995, pp 65–81

Trimble M: Post-traumatic stress disorder: history of a concept, in Trauma and Its Wake, Vol I: The Study and Treatment of Post-Traumatic Stress Disorder. Edited by Figley CR. New York, Brunner/Mazel, 1985, pp 5–14

True WR, Rice J, Eisen SA, et al: A twin study of genetic and environmental contributions to liability for posttraumatic stress symptoms. Arch Gen Psychiatry 50(4):257–264, 1993

Turkington D, Dudley R, Warman DM, Beck AT: Cognitive-behavioral therapy for schizophrenia: a review. J Psychiatr Pract 10(1):5–16, 2004

Tyrer P, Crawford M, Mulder R, et al: The rationale for the reclassification of personality disorder in the 11th revision of the International Classification of Diseases (ICD-11). Personal Ment Health 5(4):246–259, 2011

Uher R, Zwicker A: Etiology in psychiatry: embracing the reality of poly-gene-environmental causation of mental illness. World Psychiatry 16:121–129, 2017

Vaillant GE: Adaptation to Life. Boston, MA, Little Brown, 1977

Vaillant GE: The Natural History of Alcoholism Revisited. Cambridge, MA, Harvard University Press, 1995

Vaillant GE: Triumphs of Experience: The Men of the Harvard Grant Study. Cambridge, MA, Harvard University Press, 2012

Valenstein ES: Great and Desperate Cures: The Rise and Decline of Psychosurgery and Other Radical Treatments for Mental Illness. New York, Basic Books, 1988

Vassos E, Di Forti M, Coleman J, et al: An examination of polygenic score risk prediction in individuals with first-episode psychosis. Biol Psychiatry 81(6):470–477, 2017

Vidal-Ribas P, Stringaris A, Rück C, et al: Are stressful life events causally related to the severity of obsessive-compulsive symptoms? A monozygotic twin difference study. Eur Psychiatry 30(2):309–316, 2015

Wadsworth M, Kuh D, Richards M, Hardy R: Cohort profile: the 1946 National Birth Cohort (MRC National Survey of Health and Development). Int J Epidemiol 35(1):49–54, 2006

Wakefield JC, Lorenzo-Luaces L, Lee JJ: Taking people as they are: evolutionary psychopathology, uncomplicated depression, and distinction between normal and disordered sadness, in Evolutionary Psychology: The Evolution of Psychopathology. Edited by Shackelford TK and Zeigler-Hill V. New York, Springer, 2017, pp 37–72

Walker EF, Savoie T, Davis D: Neuromotor precursors of schizophrenia. Schizophr Bull 20(3):441–451, 1994

Walker FO: Huntington's disease. Lancet 369(9557):218–228, 2007

Wang J, Wu X, Lai W, et al: Prevalence of depression and depressive symptoms among outpatients: a systematic review and meta-analysis. BMJ Open 7(8):e017173, 2017

Wang J-C, Kapoor M, Goate AM: The genetics of substance dependence. Annu Rev Genomics Hum Genet 13:241–261, 2012

Ward P: Lamarck's Revenge: How Epigenetics Is Revolutionizing Our Understanding of Evolution's Past and Present. New York, Bloomsbury, 2018

Watkins LE, Sprang KR, Rothbaum BO: Treating PTSD: a review of evidence-based psychotherapy interventions. Front Behav Neurosci 12:258, 2018

Wazana A, Moss E, Jolicoeur-Martineau A, et al: The interplay of birth weight, dopamine receptor D4 gene (DRD4), and early maternal care in the prediction of disorganized attachment at 36 months of age. Dev Psychopathol 27 (4 Pt 1):1145–1161, 2015

Weaver ICG, Cervoni N, Champagne FA, et al: Epigenetic programming by maternal behavior. Nat Neurosci 7(8):847–854, 2004

Weinberger DR: Implications of normal brain development for the pathogenesis of schizophrenia. Arch Gen Psychiatry 44(7):660–669, 1987

Weissman MM, Klerman GL: Gender and depression. Trends Neurosci 8(9):416–420, 1985

Werner EE, Smith RS: Overcoming the Odds: High Risk Children From Birth to Adulthood. Ithaca, NY, Cornell University Press, 1992

White CN, Gunderson JG, Zanarini MC, Hudson JI: Family studies of borderline personality disorder: a review. Harv Rev Psychiatry 11(1):8–19, 2003

Widiger TA, Costa PT Jr (eds): Personality Disorders and the Five-Factor Model of Personality, 3rd Edition. Washington, DC, American Psychological Association, 2013

Widom CS: The cycle of violence. Science 244(4901):160–166, 1989

Widom CS: Posttraumatic stress disorder in abused and neglected children grown up. Am J Psychiatry 156(8):1223–1229, 1999

Widom CS, Czaja SJ, Paris J: A prospective investigation of borderline personality disorder in abused and neglected children followed up into adulthood. J Pers Disord 23(5):433–446, 2009

Wilkinson RG, Pickett K: The Spirit Level: Why More Equal Societies Almost Always Do Better. London, Allen Lane, 2009

Williams RR: Nature, nurture, and family predisposition. N Engl J Med 318(12):769–771, 1988

Wilson EO: Sociobiology: The New Synthesis. Cambridge, MA, Harvard University Press, 1975

Witt SH, Streit F, Jungkunz M, et al: Genome-wide association study of borderline personality disorder reveals genetic overlap with bipolar disorder, major depression and schizophrenia. Transl Psychiatry 7(6):e1155, 2017

Wolf ME, Mosnaim AD (eds): Posttraumatic Stress Disorder: Etiology, Phenomenology, and Treatment. Washington, DC, American Psychiatric Press, 1990

World Health Organization: International Classification of Diseases, 11th Revision. Geneva, World Health Organization, 2019

Wray NR, Ripke S, Mattheisen M, et al: Genome-wide association analyses identify 44 risk variants and refine the genetic architecture of major depression. Nat Genet 50(5):668–681, 2018

Yang F, Ramsay JE, Schultheiss OC, Pang JS: Need for achievement moderates the effect of motive-relevant challenge on salivary cortisol changes. Motiv Emot 39(3):321–334, 2015

Yehuda R: Post-traumatic stress disorder. N Engl J Med 346(2):108–14, 2002

Yehuda R, Lehrner A: Intergenerational transmission of trauma effects: putative role of epigenetic mechanisms. World Psychiatry 17(3):243–257, 2018

Yehuda R, Daskalakis NP, Lehrner A, et al: Influences of maternal and paternal PTSD on epigenetic regulation of the glucocorticoid receptor gene in Holocaust survivor offspring. Am Psychiatry 171(8):872–880, 2014

Young A: The Harmony of Illusions: Inventing Post-Traumatic Stress Disorder. Princeton, NJ, Princeton University Press, 1995

Zanarini MC (ed): Borderline Personality Disorder. New York, Taylor & Francis, 2005

Zheutlin AB, Dennis J, Linnér RK, et al: Penetrance and pleiotropy of polygenic risk scores for schizophrenia in 106,160 patients across four health care systems. Am J Psychiatry 176(10):846–855, 2019

Zimmerman M, Mattia J: Differences between clinical and research practices in diagnosing borderline personality disorder. Am J Psychiatry 156:1570–1574, 1999

Zimmerman M, Chelminski I, Young D: The frequency of personality disorders in psychiatric patients. Psychiatr Clin North Am 31(3):405–420, 2008

Zimmermann J, Kerber A, Rek K, et al: A brief but comprehensive review of research on the alternative DSM-5 model for personality disorders. Curr Psychiatry Rep 21(9):92, 2019

Zisook S, Kendler KS: Is bereavement-related depression different than non-bereavement-related depression? Psychol Med 37(6):779–794, 2007

Zoccolillo M, Pickles A, Quinton D, Rutter M: The outcome of childhood conduct disorder: implications for defining adult personality disorder and conduct disorder. Psychol Med 22(4):971–986, 1992

Index